Keto Diet

Stay Healthy and Live a Healthy Ketogenic Lifestyle with Simple Recipes

Tiffany Aniston

Table of Contents

Introduction

W hen your body is in a normal dietary state, it burns energy from various sources, of which three of them are the main: carbohydrates, proteins, and fats. The ketogenic diet is a diet that is very high in fat and very low in carbohydrates, with moderate consumption of protein. The reason behind the removal of carbs from the daily diet is because the body's remaining carbohydrate stores are quickly utilized for energy consumption. After they are used, the body starts to find an alternative fuel source – fat.

It is a specially formulated diet which, on the surface, appears that you will have to let go of everything you've eaten ever since your childhood; but when you dig deeper, you will understand that unlike other types of diet, the Ketogenic Diet is, well, different! It is different because it works. In general explanation of the term, a ketogenic diet is any form of dieting on food that causes the liver to produce ketones. A Ketogenic diet shifts the body's energy-burning mechanism away from glucose, to fat.

Living a Keto lifestyle is possible for you, as long as you know about the diet and what you can and can't eat. The Ketogenic diet has revived the hope of individuals who are on the verge of giving up on their weight-loss routine. This type of diet is unique. In a sense, it works on low carb diet composition. However, it doesn't put you in starving mode because you will simply replace most carbohydrates with fat, vitamins, and some proteins. The main reason why you find it difficult to lose weight is that your body has been conditioned to rely on carbs for energy. Carbs can be hard to break down in the body's system, and the fact that they slow down your metabolism simply means your weight loss will be ridiculously slow. The Ketogenic weight-loss diet works on a simple rule, and that is, to switch your body from carbohydrate-reliant to fat-burning mode. When your body enters into ketosis (the specific body condition with a keto diet), it uses up fat instead of carbs. That means your body will burn fat faster than when it is on carb-burning mode. This book has comprehensive information about the ketogenic diet that will supercharge your weight-loss journey!

Chapter 1:
The Ketogenic Diet - The Essentials

To put it in simple terms, the Keto or ketogenic diet is a diet in which you eat a very low amount of carbohydrates, and instead emphasize the consumption of a high-fat diet to produce energy for the body. By following this diet, a user can put his or her body into a state of ketosis. In this chapter, we will go deeper into what it means to produce the body's energy in this way, as opposed to other diets, as well as what a state of ketosis suggests.

Understanding Carbs.

Around the world, it is not uncommon for carbohydrates to make up most or about half of a person's daily dietary consumption. If we take a moment to look at what is the standard for an American diet, in particular, regular recommendations will ask that carbohydrates comprise a percentage of as low as 45 and up to 65 percent of your total calories on a day-to-day basis (USDA, 2015). For example, if we assume you take in about 2,000 calories a day, it would mean that anywhere from 900 to 1,300 of your daily calories would derive from carbs, which would translate to anywhere from 200 up to 325 grams of carbs in a single day.

After consumption and during the digestive process, the carbohydrates will break down and be converted into sugar, in the forms of fructose and glucose. It is then the job of the small intestines to absorb the glucose and fructose and assist in getting them into the bloodstream, which will then carry the sugars to the liver. Once in the liver, the fructose will go through a process of conversion that will turn it into glucose. It is then, with the assistance of the body's insulin, that the glucose from the liver is carried back into the bloodstream and distributed throughout the body to provide energy. This energy is used for everything from physical exertion, whether it is a walk or a heavy workout, to ensuring that you are breathing.

11

In the case that your body is not in immediate need of the glucose, the glucose will then be stored. The body stores unneeded glucose as glycogen, primarily in the skeletal muscles, and in the liver as well. Storing the glucose this way, the body will be able to hold onto about 2,000 calories worth of glycogen. If the storage of glycogen reaches a point over 2,000 calories, the body will begin to store the carbohydrates moving through your body as fat instead.

Glucose is made from the carbohydrates that you eat. Glucose is made possible as your pancreas produces the insulin needed to transport the glucose into your bloodstream, which then transports it to your cells to use for energy in various parts of the body. This same insulin is responsible for signaling the liver and the muscle tissues that it is time to save extra glucose, as well as informing the liver when the body can no longer store more glucose.

Occasionally, the liver can have a difficult time verifying that the insulin is handled appropriately and more insulin becomes needed to achieve a job. The pancreas reacts, thus creating a surge in the levels of insulin in your body to ensure that your levels of blood sugar don't become unbalanced. But rarely is this enough to secure that everything is taken care of, so excess levels of glucose often become left in your bloodstream. As a result, you experience a sudden boost of energy while eating, but end up feeling tired soon after, when you will experience a sudden drop in energy.

None of this energy fluctuation is an issue after you have accustomed your body to the keto diet, and use fat as your primary source of energy. The body becomes so efficient at burning off the extra fat, that soon it will burn off the extra body fat that is hanging around your body as well.

Why Fat Is Better

Following the Standard American Diet or SAD means that the average person takes in somewhere around 220 grams of carbohydrates in a single day, as opposed to a ketogenic diet which restricts carb intake to an absolute maximum of 50 grams per day (USDA, 2018), and even then it only applies for those whose bodies can handle it effectively. Before long, your body will have adapted to your new diet and will become a lean, mean, fat-burning machine!

No longer will you rely on carbohydrates and glucose to fuel you. Instead of storing all the excess away into fat, where it sits unused and gathering, that store will be used as your body attunes itself to using fat as its primary energy source. The levels of blood sugar in your body will not be fluctuating via booming spikes, only to plummet moments later, but it will be able to maintain a constant and steady flow of energy, which will last you all day.

So, if you're no longer taking in a high amount of carbohydrates as a part of your daily diet, then how does all this change occur from starting a high-fat, ketogenic diet? Even once your body has stopped depending on, or even being able to rely on, the consumption of carbohydrates to get glucose, it will still produce energy but will have to turn to the stores of fat to achieve it.

These stored fats will go to the liver: and once there, the fats will be broken down into glucose, and as a byproduct of the liver working with fat, the substances which we call ketones, or ketone bodies are produced. The three ketones which are formed from this process are acetate, acetoacetate, and a ketone known as BHB, which is shorthand for beta-hydroxybutyrate. These ketones, once created, act as your body's primary source of energy for activating the body in what is known as a state of ketosis.

Beta-hydroxybutyrate, it ought to be noted, is not technically known as a ketone. However, despite its slightly different chemical structure, because of its role when it comes to the Keto diet, it is commonly regarded as a ketone anyway. When the liver breaks down fat and ketogenesis is taking place, the first of the ketones to be produced is acetoacetate, which then forms into either BHB or acetone, though the acetone is a randomly-created side effect of the acetoacetate process. Despite the simple nature of acetone, it is used to transport energy through the body, although it is used very sparsely compared to BHB. Once it is no longer needed for the body's energy, it is broken down and will be removed via urine or breathing. For this reason, acetone is what is behind the commonly noted fruity smell of someone's breath who is on the ketogenic diet.

Common Keto Misconceptions

<u>Potential dangers associated with ketosis:</u> Assuming you discuss your particular needs with a healthcare provider and stick to the recommended guidelines, there is no reason that your time spent on the keto diet shouldn't be largely risk-free. With that being said, however, there are some issues you should be aware of so that you can move forward fully aware of just what you are endeavoring.

A potential issue is the fact that the keto diet can lead to low blood sugar, early on in the transition process, which means that it can be a risky proposition for those with diabetes who do not have it under control. This risk is because carbs are a common means of helping to control blood sugar levels, and many of the most common low-blood-sugar cures are carb-based. While there is research that suggests the diet might be relatively benign for those with type 2 diabetes, the risk of low blood sugar is still present.

Additionally, for those without the willpower to maintain it, the keto diet could lead to eventual "yoyo dieting". As the weight is likely to come back if you don't keep up your good eating habits, it can easily promote "yoyo dieting" which is a problem, as regaining weight may lead to other negative effects. Specifically, "yoyo dieting" in the long-term can lead to an increase of stubborn abdominal fat as well as an increased risk of diabetes. Generally speaking, the ability to stick to a diet is more important in the long-run than the type of diet you choose to follow. This rule means that if you are having a hard time following the keto diet, then it may not be for you.

Who Can and Can't Use It?

Generally speaking, if you are in good health and don't have any extenuating circumstances, then you can get started on the keto diet without delay. However, Pappas (2018) cautions that many individuals should speak with a primary healthcare provider before they get started, to ensure they don't accidentally end up doing more harm than good, such as in the following situations:

- Those who are already considered underweight, or feel as though they might have an eating disorder.

- Anyone under 18 years of age.

- Women who are pregnant or breastfeeding.

- Anyone who is recovering from a prolonged illness or serious injury.

- Those with a history of serious mental issues.

- Those with kidney issues.

- Those who are taking medications that impair liver or kidney function.

- Women who have previously had issues with irregular periods.

- Anyone with a chronic respiratory condition.

Chapter 2:
The Benefits of the Keto Diet

O f course, we can't go on with this book, without telling you what you stand to gain from the Keto Diet! The Keto diet offers a lot of benefits, ranging from weight loss to an even longer life. Of course, the level of effects will differ between individuals, but there are a few certainties, and you can be sure you have something to gain from it.

A few of the keto diet's benefits include:

Anti-Aging Capabilities

After you stop eating so many carbs, you reduce insulin formation, which in turn reduces oxidative stress, one of the factors which is responsible for human aging. Less oxidative stress means slower aging and less age-related deterioration. The ketogenic diet won't cause you to be immortal, but cutting carbs could extend your life.

Lower Blood Pressure

High blood pressure or hypertension is also called "the silent killer" because it presents no outward signs for many people. The keto diet helps to lower blood pressure.

Muscle Workout Endurance

If you wish to create muscle and train hard, the ketogenic diet can help. Naturally high in protein and healthy fats, the ketogenic diet provides your muscles with exactly what they need to grow. A high intake of healthy fats also will boost anabolic or muscle-building hormone production – namely testosterone and STH. If you wish to induce more from your gym workouts, going Keto can help.

Suppresses Appetite

Hunger is the biggest reason behind diet failure, and may undermine even the strongest willpower! When hunger strikes, it's only a matter of time before you quit your diet and give in to cravings. Low carb diets are consistently shown to provoke less hunger and ensure better dietary compliance. This, of course, ends up in faster, more sustainable, and more comfortable weight loss.

Lowers Risk of CHD

Coronary cardiovascular disease (CHD) is commonly related to a high fat intake. However, newer research suggests that it is refined carbs and sugar that are the main reason behind high blood pressure, elevated triglycerides, low "good" cholesterol, and other problems linked to CHD. Drastically reducing carbs in your diet can lessen or perhaps reverse your risk of coronary heart disease – the leading reason behind death in the USA.

Less Heartburn

Heartburn is a result of acidity within the stomach and esophagus. After just one week or two of ketogenic dieting, the general public reports less heartburn, without resorting to antacids and other heartburn medications.

Migraine Prevention

Those who suffer from migraines report suffering fewer and less severe headaches after switching from a standard diet to a ketogenic diet. There is a vital link between eating plenty of sugar and carbs, and the frequency and severity of migraine headaches.

Lowers Risk of Alzheimer's and Parkinson's disease

These diseases affect the brain and system functions, often resulting in disability and loss of independence. Studies suggest that adopting a ketogenic diet can slow the progression of those diseases and even prevent them. In addition to preventing diseases of the brain, ketogenic diets are reported to promote mental clarity, increase memory, and improve cognition.

Acne Prevention

Eating a lot of sweets can cause you to develop spots, and sugar is simply one type of carbohydrate. Low carb and ketogenic diets can help prevent acne and reduce the severity of existing outbreaks. Going Keto might also help with other skin conditions, including psoriasis and eczema.

Better Energy Levels

Most people suffer from widely fluctuating energy levels, mainly because they get their energy from carbs. In Ketosis, your body gets its energy from ketones, which it makes from fat. This means there's an almost unlimited amount of energy available, and so you're less likely to experience fluctuating energy levels and hunger between meals.

Improved Cholesterol and Triglyceride Levels

Despite being high in fat, keto diets have been shown to extend "good" cholesterol, lower "bad" LDL cholesterol, and reduce blood triglyceride profiles, all of which can reduce your risk of cardiopathy and metabolic syndrome.

Reduced Visceral Fat

Visceral or abdominal fat is stored around the internal organs and is what many doctors call "heart attack fat". It's one of the reasons your waist measurement is such a critical health indicator. Ketogenic diets are shown to be a suitable means to target visceral fat preferentially, reducing the danger of heart disease and type-2 diabetes in the process.

Chapter 3:
How to Start - for Beginners

Watch Your Macros

To get started with the keto diet successfully, the first step you need to understand involves the "macros" of the food you are eating. Macros is a shorthand term used to represent "macronutrients". These macronutrients or macros are the components we get from food, that make sure we can give energy to the body. These macros come as a result of consuming calories in the form of carbohydrates, protein, and especially for the keto diet, fats. Being able to measure and keep track of your macros is important for the ketogenic diet, because it indicates how you will know what ratio of carbs, protein, and fat your body will continue to need. This will ensure that it remains able to use fat for energy in a stable and healthy way.

Fats:

At the heart of any keto diet, despite how much you are eating, involves healthy fat foods. For your body to keep itself in a state of ketosis, you will have to make sure that it is breaking down fatty acids for its fuel, rather than carbs and glucose. For this purpose, the general recommendation is that 60 to 70, sometimes 80 percent of your daily calories should be healthy fats (Rudy Mawer, 2018). To have a keto diet that is of good quality for your mind and body, the food you are putting into it will need to be of good quality as well.

The wonderful fact about good fat foods is that they are not only good at pleasing the appetite, but also taste amazing! For what appears to be a severely restricted diet from the outset, it offers many foods to choose from, and meals to make that are as much a delicacy as they are filling. When it comes to filling out your keto diet, there are four primary types of fat for you to focus on. These are:

- saturated fats
- fats that include omega-3, which are polyunsaturated fats
- monounsaturated fats
- and only natural trans-fats.

Balancing a healthy amount of the omegas -3 and -6 is required and highly recommended, to keep your health stabilized in general. This equilibrium will keep the function of your brain and the nerves within it balanced, as well as reducing your risk of suffering heart diseases and Alzheimer's disease.

Despite the critical nature of omega-6 to your diet, having too much of it will cause inflammation in the body, so you do not want to find a source that is too high in it. Good foods for watching this are peanuts, and it will also help to make sure you are cooking your meals with corn or sunflower oil. Your source for omega-3 should be primarily from fish. Tuna and salmon are fantastic go-to options for accomplishing this goal, or you can supplement your meals with a fish oil supplement. And before we get too far away from healthy fats, be careful which nuts and seeds you are consuming, as many of them can contain high amounts of carbohydrates...

When it comes to keeping dairy in a keto diet, it is done so because it can be included as both foods that are high in fat, as well as a food that provides your body with protein. The exclusion of dairy from your diet will be rather limited, provided that you are not someone going into a keto diet, who is heavily intolerant to lactose. As with anything else, always go for the products which you know to be organic, raw, and full of fat-content.

You want your body in ketosis, so then you want your body to be able to maintain that state of ketosis. In essence, strive to ensure that you are buying and consuming dairy products that are high in protein, and contain mostly fat: these recommendations are the key when it comes

21

to adding dairy to your diet on a day-to-day basis. The dairy products that you want to be cautious of are low fat, and skimmed milk, yogurt that is low in fat, string cheese (e.g. cured mozzarella), and as with everything, avoid processed goods.

Protein:

No matter which diet you select, it is pretty important to make sure that you are getting plenty of protein in some form. There are amino acids in the protein that will keep your body regulating your organs and building muscle, as well as building connective tissue. If you can calculate your lean body mass, for which there are plenty of online resources to assist, what you want to do is eat an amount of protein that equates to about 0.8 grams of protein for each pound (455 grams) of that total number of lean body mass. While it is generally recommended on a keto diet that protein makes up around 10 to 15 percent of your total calories, you can eat more than that in protein and not put your body out of ketosis. If anyone tells you that will be too much protein, and that it will end up raising your levels of blood glucose and decreasing the levels of ketone bodies, he or she is spreading a myth.

There is a commonly misunderstood process that takes place in the body, known as gluconeogenesis or GNG for short (Brenda Godinez, 2018). Besides, there are poorly researched sources out there which claim boldly that too much protein in your keto diet will activate the GNG, elevating the levels of blood sugar in your body and ending your ketosis state. Whereas, if it were not for GNG, getting into a state of ketosis would hardly be a possibility. Ketones are incredible at many functions and especially as a source of energy, but even ketone bodies cannot be responsible for dishing out energy to 100 percent of your body tissues, which is where GNG steps in and helps the ketones to get the energy to the parts of your body that ketones alone will miss. Just as well, GNG takes place at a steady rate and will do so no matter how many amino acids are present.

When it comes to protein as well, it will likely not surprise you at this point to learn that where you get the protein from and the quality of it is as critical as the protein itself, if not more so. You want to get the highest quality meat and eggs that are within your budget. If it is grass-fed, organic, and raised on pasture, even better. And when it comes to buying a cut of meat, you want it to be on the fatty side, not too lean.

If you would like to know the highest recommended foods for filling your keto diet protein quota, they are beef (again, the fatty cuts that you can find of steak, veal, and ground beef/mince). Chicken, duck, turkey, and anything that would be considered wild is preferable. Again, still, with these, you want meat that is dark and fatty. For pork, you want it to be the loin, tenderloin, bacon, ground pork, pork chops, and ham. The animal organs are a fantastic source as well, in the form of hearts, liver, tongue, offal, etc. It is important not to forget lamb and goat meat as options.

You want to verify that you are not excluding fish from the protein portion of your diet. Tuna and salmon were mentioned earlier, there are also cod, halibut, mackerel, trout, mahi-mahi, catfish, and the list continues. You also want to include shellfish like oysters, clams, mussels, as well as crab and lobster. Delicious! There is no style of making eggs that is not recommended eating for a keto diet, just be sure to use and eat all of the egg!

Be certain you are keeping away from meats that are cured or processed, as with everything else. These come with a bunch of additives, are made with a host of chemicals, and worse, sugar. Breaded meats are important to stay away from as well, as their consumption will lead to an increase in your levels of sugars and carbohydrates.

On the keto diet, to make sure your body is in a healthy, balanced, and well-maintained state of ketosis, you will want to do your best to have your carbs come from sources like leafy vegetables, broccoli, asparagus, cauliflower, and nearly any other vegetable that is grown above the ground. The vegetables that are higher in starch will cause some trouble. You will also be getting some of your carbohydrate intakes for the day from nuts and seeds, and there will be a minuscule amount which you get from some dairy products, and an off-chance that any berries you are eating will provide a small number of carbs as well.

Carbs:

Carbohydrates are the commonest major macronutrient that comprises the food most people eat. Besides reducing carbohydrates, the keto diet is also interested in them, as well as fat and protein. Being a primary component of energy production in the body, carbs are most recognizable as starch, fiber, and sugar in the form of bread, cereals, beans, pasta, rice, and potatoes, while also occurring naturally in fruits, vegetables, and milk.

While you are only allowed a very small amount of carbs per day, this limitation doesn't mean you can blow them all off, without giving them a second thought. Instead, it is important to use your carb allotment on healthy choices like dark, leafy green vegetables as they are going to have more nutrients per serving than any other alternative.

Vegetables that have a viable number of carbs when consumed in moderation include things like kale, sprouts, garlic, cabbage, radishes, spinach, dill pickles, bok choy, broccoli, asparagus, cauliflower, chives, leeks, and cucumbers. However, if your favorite type of vegetable isn't on this list, that doesn't mean it's off-limits completely: instead, it only means that you are going to need to track carefully how much you consume, to avoid making a costly mistake.

Supplements:

The first of these supplements mentioned are exogenous ketones (Nate Arnold, 2019). The reason someone would usually utilize exogenous ketone supplements would be simply to provide extra ketones for the body. If nothing else, they are at least helpful when first starting a keto diet, for helping your body with the energy-use transition, getting you into ketosis faster, and are also a helpful way to get ketosis going and maintained while you are fasting.

If you are at a point where you would maybe have to wait a couple of days to get into a state of ketosis and would rather desire to speed up the process, then exogenous ketones are the way for you to go. Exogenous ketones are easy to take between one meal and the next, and they offer your body a swift batch of ketone bodies. They are also useful before a daily workout, as they give your body that extra bit of energy it may need.

There are also MCT or medium-chain triglycerides (Sharon O'Brien, 2018) which come in the form of an oil or powder. MCT is a kind of fat that can be utilized to give your body a ketone energy-source that does not require that it go through the digestive process, to be used. They act as a first step in the ketone process and will help your body to ensure that it is burning the fats it needs for ketosis, as opposed to carbohydrates.

The use of MCT oil or powder has several benefits. As they are easily digestible and almost immediately have the desired effect of being an alternative source of fuel, they are an incredible way of giving your metabolism a boost to lose weight. MCT oils and powders are one of the fastest-acting ways of getting the energy to the body: they are quickly broken down into ketones, and then your body can use them for fuel.

MCTs are also useful when it comes to supporting your digestive system, by offering support to your gut biome (i.e. the bacteria in your intestines) which it accomplishes by combatting the bacteria and parasites which would normally be harmful. And when it comes to your health in general, MCT oil and powder deliver a host of antioxidant properties which are primed for reducing any inflammation you may have internally, and assisting the functioning of your nervous system, your brain, and even your heart.

Our third option for supplementing ketosis is collagen protein. Protein, in the form of collagen, makes up one of the over 10.000 proteins in your body. Of all these proteins though, collagen is the one which is most prevalent, making up 25 to 35 percent of all of the protein in your body (Genetics Home Reference, 2019). If you would like to think of it in this way, you could imagine it as a glue keeping the rest of your body held together.

When it comes in the form of beef which is grass-fed, collagen is produced the same way that you would go about preparing a bone-broth, with a slow cooking process over low heat, which is intended to preserve the nutritional content. The health of your organs needs to keep collagen as a key component of your keto diet. It is also useful in maintaining the health of your muscles, joints, eyes, hair, nails, skin, and heart.

Don't Forget Fat Bombs

After you have removed practically all of the carbohydrates from your diet, you are likely to feel a carbohydrate-sized hole in your diet, especially when it comes to grabbing a quick snack, or looking for something to provide a quick burst of energy! In the world of the keto diet, the role of the in-between meal snack is known as a "fat bomb". A fat bomb is a quick-to-eat snack that can be either sweet or savory, and is full of healthy fats from items like butter, coconut oil, seeds, and nuts, which means they are often 80 or 90 percent healthy fat per serving.

Not only will the energy in these snacks get you up and moving, but the healthy fats will also fill you up and satiate you until your next proper meal comes around. Even better, it will do both of these things in a way that is much more effective than the carbohydrate-filled fashion to which you are likely already accustomed. This lack of carbs means they are the perfect choice if you are planning to go to the gym, or know you won't have time to fix yourself a healthy dinner until later than normal. What's more, they will help you to get your daily allotment of fats each day, which is going to be more difficult some days than you might expect.

While fat bombs can be a quick, easy, and, most importantly, healthy option to round out your diet, that doesn't mean they shouldn't still be consumed in moderation, especially at first. It is important to keep in mind that your body might have an initially poor reaction to so much fat, whether healthy or not, so you will want to introduce all your new dietary rules over a week or so to ensure that your body doesn't have any other major dietary concerns to consider, while it is making the difficult transition to ketosis.

The Four Phases of a Proper Keto Diet

The four phases of the keto diet reflect the changes in energy requirements you need as you eventually go from weight loss all the way to weight maintenance. Don't forget, the keto diet is a lifestyle more than it is a traditional diet, which means that once you make the change, you should plan to settle in for the long-term for the best results.

1. Induction phase:
The first phase, known as the induction phase, will account for the first few weeks of your time spent with the keto diet. After your body gets over the "keto flu", this period is when you are likely to see the greatest amount of weight loss per week. During this period, you can expect your body fat to provide up to 50 percent of all of the caloric energy your body is using per day.

While the keto diet doesn't require any calorie restriction in its base form, successfully making it past the "keto flu" and into ketosis for the first time is likely to cause a decrease in appetite naturally, which is a benefit to maintaining a steady level of blood sugar over a prolonged period. This process is also part of the reason the body burns extra fat during this period as well. The body will use as many as 200 grams of fat per day for energy during this period, which means you need to ensure your fat intake is as high as possible and your carb intake is as low as possible, to ensure your body makes the transition as fully and effectively as possible.

2. Weight -oss phase:
The next phase is known as the weight-loss phase. While your body is in it, your body fat will continue to decrease though not as quickly as it did during the previous phase. During this period, it is common for total caloric consumption to increase by a few hundred calories per day, but total caloric deficit should be maintained relatively easily thanks to the amount of fat the body is still burning naturally. It is normal for carb intake to increase slightly during this period, though the total net carbs should not increase much, if at all. The same is true for protein. By this time, body fat is typically providing about a third of all daily energy needs, which are decreasing by the day as body weight decreases.

3. Pre-maintenance phase:
During the pre-maintenance phase, you will see your weight loss begin to slow down even more, as your body has exhausted most of your existing fat stores so that the caloric deficit you are running daily will decrease even more. It is a natural part of the process, however, as it is usual to settle eventually into an extended weight loss phase, where you will lose about one pound of fat per week. Indeed, it is considered a healthy norm for extended weight loss.

4. Maintenance phase:
As the name suggests, during this phase all body fat stores have been exhausted, and the goal of the keto diet changes. It stops being about losing existing weight, and becomes more about sticking with the lifestyle in such a way that you don't need to worry about excessive weight gain in the future. Carb intake can typically increase by about 10 grams in this phase, though you may be able to add more or less back in, depending on your body. Experiment with various combinations and see what works for you.

"Keto Flu"

Once you've decided to adopt a ketogenic lifestyle, it is important to be aware of the fact that a state of ketosis will not be achieved after you skip a couple of low carb meals. Rather, if you proceed down this path, you will find that it will take as many as 7 days before you start to feel the effects of ketosis. Be warned: the interim period is likely to be rough going, as your body will be burning through all of its fuel reserves without having the benefit of ketones to pick up the slack. During this period, it is extremely important to stick to your guns, as cutting out carbohydrates slowly will only prolong your suffering.

Forewarned is forearmed, however, and there are a few measures you can take to encourage your body to enter ketosis as quickly and easily as possible. First things first: if you are exercising regularly, make sure you are doing so on an empty stomach, as it will further reduce the leftover glucose in your body. Likewise, you may also find that skipping an extra meal here or there will get you to where you need to be more quickly. Essentially, any time your stomach is growling is a period that is actively pushing you towards a state of ketosis. Finally, during this period you are going to want to stick to a strict limit of 20 grams of carbohydrates per day, or less, to get you to where you need to be.

While preparing to enter ketosis, it is also possible you will experience some of the following side effects. It is important to keep in mind that not all who take on the keto diet are guaranteed to experience all, or even any, of the side effects that it's possible to go through. But the keto diet is not for everyone, unfortunately. There may be ways for you to work around it and make it work for you, but that is something you will have to discuss with your doctor or a dietary professional, to make sure you are doing it in a way that maximizes your potential and the benefits that you are getting from the diet.

Dehydration:

When entering ketosis, your body will be much more efficient at burning off the glucose stored in your liver and muscles, doing so very quickly even within the first couple of days of starting the diet. This process means that you will be releasing a lot of water. Your kidneys will also start to excrete more sodium than normal during this time, due to the levels of insulin you have circulating starting to drop. As a result, it is more than likely that you may notice you need to stop and go to the restroom more often to pee during the day. This small side effect will come right by itself, though, once your body has become accustomed to the new way of working.

Excess of flu symptoms:

In the first few days of taking on the keto lifestyle as a diet plan, you may exhibit what is a common side effect known as the "keto flu" or even has been called "induction flu". It is named so because the symptoms of keto flu resemble those of the actual flu. You may find you have a headache, some lethargy, and a lack of motivation; your brain may feel a bit foggy and unclear, and, or, you also become a bit more irritable.

As with the increased frequency of urination, these symptoms will go away completely on their own, and in just a few days, once your body is more in line and used to using ketones for its source of energy, and you are in ketosis mode. The keto flu and its symptoms are also pretty easy to avoid if you can keep yourself drinking plenty of water, as well as trying to hike it up a little bit on the amount of salt that you are consuming. And, as it goes with the keto diet in general, no matter what the case may be, be sure to eat plenty of healthy fats.

Acetone discharge:

The acetone that is created during the ketosis process can be expelled from the body when it is not needed, and this is through waste, via the urine, or by leaving the body when you exhale. It is not at all uncommon to hear from people that the smell of the acetone is lingering in their breath once they have begun eating a low carb diet and their body has adapted to being in ketosis. The acetone has been noted as sometimes giving breath a fruity smell, or even sometimes a smell that could be compared to nail polish remover. Although people may comment on this to you, it is a sign that you are in a state of ketosis, which is the goal. Your body is busy burning off all of the healthy fats you are eating, and is processing them into the ketone bodies you need to keep energized, all according to plan.

When this symptom has been noticed in people, typically it tends to be something that goes away nearly as quickly as it began. In short, it usually happens within a few days to a week, and then leaves again in just a week or two. If the body can adapt fully into being in a state of ketosis regularly, it will subdue a lot of the early symptoms of the diet. If you are one of the lucky ones for whom the smell happens to persist, the ideal way to correct it is by just having good hygiene when it comes to your mouth. You ought to be doing it already, but especially at this point be sure that you are brushing your teeth twice a day at the very least, as well as rinsing with some mouthwash.

This area highlights another tip for keeping the amount of water you are drinking increased, to benefit you. If you have bad breath, this side effect can be due to a lack of saliva in your mouth, which can result from your mouth becoming drier as more water is getting expelled while you are in a state of ketosis. Drinking plenty of water during the day is always suggested, and it is recommended that you drink 64 fluid ounces (2 liters) per day, despite which diet you pursue.

Testing for Ketosis

One of the most popular ways that you can measure the levels of ketones in your body is through the use of a urine strip. This tool is the most common method, simply because of its ease of access. Urine strips are generally cheap and can be found at local stores like Walgreens and CVS in the USA.

However, despite how easily they can be purchased, it is more than possible for urine strips to be low in reliability. After being on a keto diet for only a short time, your body will quickly become more attuned to this way of life and its efficiency, when it comes to producing and using ketones as energy. As a consequence it will increase drastically, and once your body has done this, ketosis has become the body's natural way of being for you. This allows it to be so efficient at energy use that using a urine strip may not be able to show the level of ketosis accurately.

The accuracy of a test done this way can also be skewed by how much you have hydrated for the day, as well as the number of electrolytes in your body at the time of taking the test. Because of these factors affecting the accuracy of your reading when using a urine strip, it is a method of measurement that is usually only a recommendation for people who are newer to the keto diet.

Just as people who check for diabetes use a blood glucose meter, you can use the same device as a method for measuring the levels of ketones in the blood, especially for the ketone BHB or beta-hydroxybutyrate. It is one of the most highly recommended ways of checking your levels on your own due to the accuracy of the testing. There are very few factors that will make an effect on the test, either in a negative or positive reading, making it one of the most reliable ways of testing your ketone levels. It does come at a slight price when compared to the urine test, as it can cost you about 5 to 10 dollars for each strip needed to test your blood in this way.

Chapter 4:
Keto Tips and Tricks for Beginners

When you are just starting the path down the road to keto eating, it can be hard to know what to get at the grocery-store and how to achieve the most bang for your buck at the same time. Organic veggies are pesticide-free, grass-fed meat is often more delicious and has superior nutrition, and free-range eggs are incredibly nutritious. However, what do all these items have in common? They are expensive. Their price point makes them an automatic scratch-off when it comes to options for those who live on a strict food budget.

If you live on fast food, diet soda, and fries, switching to regular eggs, veggies, and meat will still have a huge impact on your overall health. The vital aspect of a healthier lifestyle is to cook at home from scratch.

1. Don't Plan for Three Meals Daily

People on the keto diet are sure to go through a decrease in appetite the moment ketosis kicks in. This can ruin your planned meals in a day, as you might have to skip either lunch, breakfast, or dinner. So you shouldn't go through all the stress of planning for three meals a day.

This lack of appetite can last from a few days to up to weeks, depending on each individual, activity level, and genes. It could also be affected by your former eating habits.

2. It Helps to Add a Bit of Olive Oil or Avocado Oil to Your Meal

Olive oil contains lots of healthy fat. More often than not, people get frustrated with their keto diet because they don't get enough fat, or at least not the right kind of fat.

People make the mistake of sticking to one kind of fat, which is saturated fat. This is not the best. You have to vary your fat-consumption while on the keto diet.

You can prevent this from happening with a good addition of olive or avocado oils to your meals. Olive oil contains lots of monosaturated fatty acids, and these fats are healthy.

Avocado oil also shares this quality.

People usually consume the wrong types of fat, in excess. Examples of such fats are deli meat, fatty meats, bacon, sausage, butter, and lard. These fats can be bad for your blood pressure and heart health and may even cause digestive issues.

3. Cut Back on Protein Portions

Many believe that the keto diet is a high-protein diet, and this is not exactly true. Many believe that simply because they eat few carbs, they should automatically get into Ketosis. The fact is, other factors might be keeping you out, factors such as excess consumption of protein.

The average person on a keto diet should reduce their protein intake by half. So you go from about eating a 10-ounce (300g) steak to a 5-ounce (150g) steak.

4. Respect Your Body

The keto diet is admittedly very restrictive. It is not uncommon for beginners to get caught up in all the numbers. Sure, there are threshold numbers you have to measure up to, but it is more important to listen to what your body is telling you, and respect it.

You can start consuming less than 20 grams of net carbs (i.e. available, digestible carbs). Then you wait out the transition symptoms, which should begin to manifest after a few days. After they've come and gone, you should feel amazing.

You've got to give plenty of attention to your feelings, your mental clarity, and your energy levels. The transition will make you foggy at first, but when it ends, it will feel like a cloud has cleared up in the sky of your mind.

5. Adopt Useful Fat-Rich Sources and Go-to-Dishes

It is prevalent for people to break their diet out of boredom, because of eating the same things over again.

Avocados and eggs may taste great now, but they could seem boring quickly. So, if you know you want to commit yourself to the Keto diet, you should pick up and master a few go-to dishes, which are also rich sources of fat. You could try the lemon-cream sauce or pesto. But don't be limited; there are a lot out there to try.

6. Know the Number of Carbs in Your Veggies

Not all vegetables are suitable for the keto diet, not even all the leafy greens. You should always consider how many carbs could be in there. Sure, it may be a bit weird to measure your spinach, but it is essential to make sure you don't go over the carb limit.

There are many veggies out there that are strictly carbohydrates, whether or not they are little carbs for the total volume of food you want to eat. Simply consider your five favorite green vegetables that you eat most often, and look up how many carbs they have per serving. Now you'll always know how much you can have of each of those vegetables per meal.

The bottom line is, you need to keep track of the carbs in your veggies for you to enter Ketosis.

7. Your Health Comes First

Suppose you began the keto diet, but soon things started getting out of hand, or you were frustrated and miserable. In that case, you should reconsider your position on the keto diet. The fact is, just because a lot of people are doing it and it works for them, doesn't mean you must.

Many people have gone into this diet only on a recommendation by a friend or family member, or they hear that Beyoncé does it and decide to question their entire feeding habits. This shouldn't be the case. If it's for you, do it;but if you feel it is not, there are other ways to achieve your goals, albeit a lot longer and more difficult.

8. Don't Take Unnecessary Risks

The health and diet world is not in complete agreement with the safety of the keto diet. Some say it is unsafe and unfit for humans, yet others suggest that it will work for the right person if monitored carefully. However, you should know that there could be instances where the keto diet increases the risk of kidney issues.

Moreover, the keto diet is NOT advisable for pregnant women, or if you're trying to get pregnant. This is because the keto diet puts you at a high risk of missing essential nutrients like folate, which is essential for women trying to conceive.

So, if you plan to go the keto way and have reservations about your health, you should consult a professional. See a registered dietitian or your local health care provider, who will know more about the possible risks before you start the keto diet.

Essential principles and practical tips for a high-fat diet

1. Not All Fats Are Equally Healthy

In the same way that carbohydrates (like sugar, starch and dietary fiber) are different, so are fats.

Try to consume as many mono- and polyunsaturated fats as possible, especially those that are rich in omega acids (like coconut oil, which you can read about below). That is, refined oil, which is purely fat and nothing but fat, devoid of any other properties.

This also applies to mayonnaise, which is 90% of this oil (however, mayonnaise will now be the most important of all sauces for you). You must also be careful with cheeses - even if they are fatty and contain a tiny amount of carbohydrates (sometimes equal to nothing at all), but they are high in calories, so the process of losing weight can slow down a lot.

Eat organic or grass-fed fat beef (steaks and burgers without rolls), pork, free-range chicken with skin, generously season salad leaves (the main source of carbohydrates in the keto diet) with unrefined olive oil, and fry in ghee, which is clarified butter (or almost the same). If ghee can't be bought, do it yourself.

Do this:

- take a large package of butter (80% fat and more)
- cut into cubes
- put them in a pan
- bring to a boil

- and on the smallest fire, melt for a couple of hours until the mixture becomes uniformly golden.

And of course bacon, which is almost 100% animal fat, is the best breakfast companion.

2. Drink Plenty of Water

Two liters per day is the minimum. With a Ketogenic Diet, don't forget about it – drinking too little is dangerous for your health, and good hydration helps weight loss a lot.

There is even an opinion that water helps to keep you in ketosis, and even if you don't follow the rest of the rules but monitor the water balance, you can still achieve good results.

With Keto, a lot of the waste is removed from the body through urine, and water helps to speed this up and establish better digestion.

3. Drink 2 Cups of Broth Daily

With a Ketogenic Diet, the body might lack salts and minerals, with consequences such as cramps, muscle pain, and headaches.

Especially, headaches during adaptation - that is from the first week the body enters ketosis.

This can be avoided with the help of salt broth - it contains all the necessary minerals. You can cook it from fat chicken, drink a glass in the morning and evening - and never get sick. However, if after a couple of months, the muscles still behave strangely - take vitamins with magnesium and potassium.

4. Buy Coconut Oil

As mentioned above, with a Keto Diet, you'll need to consume as many saturated fats and fatty acids as possible - all this, in incredible amounts, is contained in coconut oil.

Plus, coconut oil has a very high combustion temperature; that is, it can be used for frying if the taste won't bother you, or you can eat some spoons of it.

5. Start the Day with "Bulletproof Coffee"

If you drink coffee, then you should drink it like this:
On a glass of Americano - a spoonful of butter, and a spoonful of coconut oil.

It sounds disgusting: but in the end, butter is made from cream, which no one seems to be shy about putting in coffee, and coconut gives it a delightful aftertaste!
This mixture is called "bulletproof coffee", and in addition to a charge of vivacity, and a whole bunch of advantages described, it also saves you from stool problems that may arise with a keto diet.

6. Snack on Nuts

The Keto-diet robs you of chips - even muesli, even chocolate bars, and in general, almost everything that you can quickly have a snack of when "on the go" and in the workplace.
There is a way out - nuts - primarily almonds, forest nuts, and cedar nuts.
If you were expecting to see cashew nuts: sorry, this isn't among them.
These nuts mentioned contain a large number of fatty acids and are moderate in dietary fiber (that is, those carbohydrates that should not be excluded entirely from the diet).
50 g of almonds contains almost 20 g of saturated fat and 10 g of carbs - and this is enough for a snack.

7. Be Careful with Sweeteners

Of course, sweets will not stop tempting you and sweeteners might seem like a way out, but they can be dangerous.

First, always check the nutritional value: for example, the most common non-sucrose sweetener, fructose, is 100% carbohydrate.

Secondly, you will never find an ideal sweetener, and you can't avoid all sorts of aftertastes. Some sweeteners may cause diarrhea in larger amounts.

Thirdly, carefully monitor the reaction of your body: sometimes, even just feeling the sweetness, the body automatically takes it for sugar and produces insulin. That could be an instant knock out, by diet cola, from ketosis. By the way, you can check whether your body is in ketosis with the help of glucose and Ketone test strips - if the piece is purple, then most likely, everything is in order. The test can be inaccurate and faulty, but is generally suitable for control.

8. Chocolate is Not to Blame for Anything

Another bit of good news is that chocolate contains incredibly healthy cocoa butter. The wrong side of this news is that in addition to this, milk chocolate also has a brutal amount of sugar; but you can buy bitter, 72% cocoa, and more. Have a couple of slices instead of sweets (they still hide 4-8 g of sugar, but with this, you can survive).

An even safer option is to buy chocolate with 99% cocoa and make truffles from it: melt, knead with butter or coconut oil, add fat cream, sweeter to taste when fresh, and roll into balls that can be decorated with either crushed almonds or coconut flakes.

One such shot will contain no more than 2 g of carbohydrates from cocoa beans and cream.

9. Look for Keto Food in the City - It's Easy

Dieting doesn't mean that now you have to eat only what you cook for yourself. You can go into any burger restaurant and eat a patty, after getting rid of the rolls! In fast foods, you can order a vegetable salad to the cutlet, and in diners - ask for a double portion of lettuce and use the mixture instead of bread.

By the way, in "Starlite" you can get such a burger, as it's on the menu and is called, 'Excuse Me, Hipster'. Remember that in "Subway" there is always the opportunity to order any of their sandwiches in a salad instead of bread.

In places where you can safely eat shawarma, you can order it on a plate. There are more and more fast-food chains offering budget steaks and a large selection of green salads - the Yummy Mix chain, for example.

In general, you can live a full life and not endure the house where the cutlet is wrapped in bacon.

10. Use the Internet

It sounds like the most idiotic advice in the world, but do you know that if you enter the name of any product in Google, for example, then right on the results page, you can see the nutritional value of this product?

This is extremely useful, for example, in queues in a cafeteria - you can understand in a minute that this broccoli is not only possible for you, but also necessary. Secondly, look for recipes. Eating eggs, bacon, steaks, and meatballs every day seems like a good idea only at first, but then you'll want variety.

Chapter 5:
The Top 10 Keto Diet Foods

N ow it's time to restock your freezer, refrigerator, and pantry with keto-friendly, delicious foods that will make you feel great, get healthy, and lose weight. Each of these 10 staples is versatile and can be incorporated into breakfast, lunch, dinner, snacks, and dessert.

#1: Butter and Ghee

Butter and ghee are often used interchangeably, even to the point that they are confused as being one and the same thing. They are different, though! Ghee is clarified butter, which is butter that has been heated until the milk solids settle to the bottom, cook and separate. There are different ways to cook it, but we usually boil it until it becomes a hard golden butter.

Why are butter and ghee great for the ketogenic diet? Note that butter is better for managing and preventing heart disease than ghee. Ghee is also used as a meditative aid, as it is said to bring about a tranquil state of mind. Both can be used for cooking, but ghee can withstand much higher temperatures than butter. Butter can be kept in the fridge for 3-4 days, while ghee can be stored properly in the freezer for a year. Upon melting, butter produces small air bubbles and tends to cook more like a solid. Having no bubbles in ghee causes it to cook more like oil. Ghee is perfect for making stir-fries and oven-roasted vegetables, and for general frying.

#2: Avocado

Unlike many other filling fruits, avocados can be used interchangeably as a topping for everything from cheese-based food to eggs. It provides healthy fats and fiber, while its heart-healthy nature is a good reason to include it in your daily diet.

Why avocado is great for the ketogenic diet: folate is an important factor in the body that makes it a heart-healthy food. Avocados are a great source of it, combined with the right fatty acids, fiber, potassium, and vitamins. Avocados also carry a good amount of vitamin E, which is an antioxidant that helps to prevent disease. The fats in the avocado act as an easy-energy food and are great for the ketogenic diet.

The best part about avocado is that, with the addition of a few spices, it can become a tasty dish for the whole family. We're aware that they might not be on your keto diet, so we're going to include some things you won't be able to eat, but which they'll love. It might convince them that they don't have to stop enjoying food if they went on your diet! Let's take a look at some of the things we can do with avocado (*note that some might not be right for you on your keto diet!):

- Guacamole – You've probably heard of guacamole – it's a dip created with avocado that's full of other tasty ingredients.
- *Crépes – Did you know that avocado is an excellent addition to pancake batter?
- *Spread – Spread avocado on bread, or add it to a sandwich, for them to enjoy!
- Smoothie – Did you know that avocado tastes great in smoothies, too? Stir it into your yogurt, just to give it that extra boost, or to mix it with some fruit.
- Sauce – You can add avocado, as well as some onion and spices, to some soup for an amazing meal! You can add this to your meat as a tasty sauce, giving flavor, and smoothness if the meat is dry.
- Mousse – You can also use your favorite full-fat yogurt as the base for a delicious avocado mousse.
- Cheese – You can use full-fat mascarpone in a wonderful topping for your avocado flavors, too. Enjoy!
- Dip – For the best dips, have some avocado as a base. You can try the guacamole, simply made with avocado or the spiced-up flavor of chipotle chilis.
- Soup – Have some gazpacho with pureéd avocado added.

- Ice cream – It's time to enjoy some home-made, nutrient-packed ice cream. Just make sure it's not high in sugar, and add pureéd avocado before freezing!
- Pasta Sauce – You can make a healthy (well, healthier) pasta with your favorite tomato sauce and avocado.
- Eggs – You can add avocado to an omelet.

#3: Cinnamon

Although not the most popular spice, it contains a chemical called "cinnam-aldehyde" which has some interesting benefits, such as aiding in weight loss by lowering the craving for calories in your meals. The spice can enhance the health and beauty of a variety of dishes.

Why cinnamon is great for the ketogenic diet: It is rich in cinnamaldehyde that can lower your appetite. It is also a great chili substitution for those who have to grill their meat. Calcium from the cinnamon is what is responsible for its cholesterol-lowering effect.

#4: Coconut Oil

This oil is high in saturated fat, but it is perfectly healthy – especially for those with high cholesterol. It has a high amount of MCTs, a type of fat that helps with body composition while also reducing hunger.

Why coconut oil is great for the ketogenic diet: It can be used as a substitution for butter and ghee, but it is especially good at carrying a rich coconut flavor. It is great for searing meats, because it has a high flashpoint. The cholesterol-lowering quality comes from its MCTs. It has also been shown to improve insulin symptoms, so it is particularly great for people with diabetes.

#5: Dark Chocolate

Yes, you read that right. Dark chocolate is a keto-friendly food item. While it contains sugar, it also has a lot of healthy cocoa that can assist with weight loss.

Why dark chocolate is great for the keto diet: Choco-Lite, a type of dark chocolate often sweetened with artificial sweeteners, is specially designed to give a sweet taste for those who want to cut down on their calorie intake. Or, any dark chocolate with 70 percent or more cocoa has less sugar, but still gives you a sweet taste. This will satisfy your hunger better than sugars would.

#6: Cottage Cheese

Yes, you also read that right. Cottage cheese is great for the ketogenic diet.
Why cottage cheese/cottage cheese curds are great for the ketogenic diet: it is a perfect snack for those on the diet. You can eat it plain, add it to something else, or make a salad, or simply eat it with a fork. It is also very low in carbs, just 1 net carb content per cup. Cottage cheese can be kept refrigerated for up to a couple of weeks with no loss of flavor, not like other brands that cannot be kept for very long.

#7: Avocado Oil

This type of oil is great for cooking at higher temperatures and is an excellent addition to many dishes. It can be used for cooking at high temperatures and is a great substitute for extra virgin olive oil.

Why avocado oil is great for the ketogenic diet: the high amount of MCTs is a big bonus for fat loss, especially for the ketogenic diet. Avocado oil is a good substitute for extra virgin olive oil, as it has a four-times-higher monounsaturated fat content ,while still having some of the fatty acids that may help to prevent heart disease. Superhealthline.com notes that avocado oil is also a good weight-loss choice, and

45

that diets low in fat and high in carbohydrates can be a major source of obesity. After all, we know avo oil is satisfying for your appetite, so that you're less likely to crave carbs.

#8: Chicken Wings

Sometimes called just "wings", chicken wings are a great addition to the ketogenic diet. They are high in protein and low in fat and carbs. Because chicken wings lack carbs, it makes them a dietary staple for any weight-loss diet.

The wings are a common item in many ketogenic meal plans, but can also be served as an appetizer – perfect for parties and social gatherings. Best of all, you don't have to spend a fortune on them, as far as the ketogenic diet goes, you can feel free in any meal.

#9: Beef or Beef Heart

Beef can be a great addition to any diet, and in the keto diet it makes sense that many people have made the switch from buying only lean cuts of steak to buying fattier cuts. Most of the time, people turn to beef when the going gets tough because it makes for a fantastic keto meal in itself as meat.

Beef is very straightforward to make into broth, and for that reason, beef broth is also a staple in a lot of people's meals. It's usually inexpensive and takes very little time to prepare – which makes it the perfect option for those looking for an easy meal.

#10: Cheese

Cheese is another amazing food keto dieters tend to enjoy. It is so versatile in many different types of meals, ranging from adding flavor to being the base of a dish. Many people do not even miss the carbs from the types of food they used to eat, as there are other alternatives, such as fatty cheeses. For example, there is Gouda, a semi-hard, full-fat cheese, that packs approximately 20 grams of carbs in every 100 grams. As far as cheeses go, this one is not too shabby. Harder cheeses such as Parmesan are excellent to add flavor to veggies, eggs, even fish.

Chapter 6:
Keto Recipes

(For metric conversion tables, see chapter 8)

Breakfast

Savory Breakfast Bowl

Preparation & Cooking time: 30 minutes
Serves: 2
Ingredients:

- 4 ounces hamburger, ground/minced
- One yellow onion, chopped
- Eight mushrooms, sliced
- Salt and black pepper to taste
- Two eggs, whisked
- One tablespoon coconut oil
- ½ teaspoon smoked paprika
- One avocado, de-stoned, peeled, and chopped
- 12 dark olives, de-stoned and sliced

Directions:

1. Heat up a saucepan with the coconut oil over medium warmth, include onion, mushrooms, salt, and pepper, mix and cook for 5 min.

2. Include meat and paprika, mix, cook for 10 min, and move to a bowl.

3. Heat up the saucepan again over medium warmth, include eggs, some salt and pepper, and scramble them.

4. Return meat blend to dish and mix. Include avocado and olives, mix and cook for a few moments.

5. Move to bowls and serve.

6. Relax and enjoy it!

Nourishment: calories 600.Grams: fat 23, fiber 8, carbs 22, protein 43.

Delectable Eggs and Sausages

Prep & Cooking time: 45 minutes
Serves: 6
Ingredients:
- Five tablespoons ghee
- 12 eggs
- Salt and black pepper to taste
- 1 ounce spinach, shredded
- 12 ham slices
- Two frankfurters chopped
- One yellow onion chopped
- One red bell pepper chopped

Directions:
1. Heat up a frying-pan with 1-tablespoon ghee over medium warmth, include frankfurters and onion, mix and cook for 5 min.
2. Include bell pepper, salt, and pepper, mix and cook for 3 min more and move to a bowl.
3. Dissolve the remainder of the ghee and pour into 12 cupcake molds.
4. Include a slice of ham in every cupcake form, separate spinach in each, and afterward, the frankfurter blend.
5. Break an egg on top, put everything in the stove and cook at 425 degrees F for 20 min.
6. Leave your Keto cupcakes to chill off a bit before serving on the plate.
7. Relax and enjoy!

Nourishment: calories 440. Grams: fat 32, fiber 10, carbs 12, protein 22

Fried Eggs

Prep & Cooking time: 20 minutes
Serves: 2
Ingredients:

- Four button mushrooms, chopped
- Three eggs, whisked
- Salt and black pepper to taste
- Two ham slices, chopped
- ¼ cup red bell pepper, chopped
- ½ cup spinach, chopped
- One tablespoon coconut oil

Directions:

1. Heat up a dish with half of the oil over medium warmth, include mushrooms, spinach, ham, and bell pepper, mix and cook for 4 min.
2. Heat up another dish with the remainder of the oil over medium warmth, include eggs, and scramble them.
3. Include veggies and ham, salt and pepper, mix, cook for a few moments, and serve.

Relax and enjoy!
Nourishment: calories 350. Grams: fat 23, fiber 1, carbs 5, protein 22.

Delectable Frittata

Prep & Cooking: 1 hour 10 minutes
Serves: 4
Ingredients:

- 9 ounces spinach
- 12 eggs
- 1-ounce pepperoni
- One teaspoon garlic, minced
- Salt and black pepper to taste
- 5 ounces mozzarella, grated
- ½ cup parmesan, ground
- ½ cup ricotta cheddar
- Four tablespoons olive oil
- A pinch of nutmeg

50

Directions:

1. Crush fluid from spinach and put it in a bowl.

2. In another bowl, blend eggs with salt, pepper, nutmeg, and garlic and whisk well.

3. Include spinach, parmesan, and ricotta and whisk well once more.

4. Empty this into an oven tray, sprinkle mozzarella and pepperoni on top, put into the oven, and heat at 375 degrees F for 45 min.

5. Leave frittata to chill off for a couple of moments before plating it. Relax and enjoy!

Nourishment: calories 298.Grams: fat 2, fiber 1, carbs 6, protein 18.

Smoked Salmon Breakfast

Prep & Cooking time: 20 minutes
Serves: 3
Ingredients:

- Four eggs whisked
- ½ teaspoon avocado oil
- 4 ounces smoked salmon, chopped

For the sauce:

- 1 cup of coconut milk
- ½ cup cashews, crushed
- ¼ cup green onions, chopped
- One teaspoon garlic powder
- Salt and black pepper to taste
- One tablespoon lemon juice

Directions:

1. In your blender, blend cashews in coconut milk, garlic powder, and lemon juice and mix well.

2. Place salt, pepper, and green onions; mix again well, move to a bowl, and keep in the cooler until later.

3. Heat up a container with the oil over medium-low warmth, include eggs, whisk a little and cook until they are nearly done.

4. Put in your preheated oven and cook until eggs set.

5. Put eggs on plates, top with smoked salmon, and serve with the green onion sauce on top.

Relax and enjoy!

Nourishment: calories 200. Grams: fat 10, fiber 2, carbs 11, protein 15.

Feta and Asparagus Delight

Prep & Cooking time: 35 minutes

Serves: 2

Ingredients:

- 12 asparagus spears
- One tablespoon olive oil
- Two green onions, chopped
- One garlic clove, minced
- Six eggs
- Salt and black pepper to taste
- ½ cup feta cheese (you can substitute with cheddar)

Directions:

1. Heat up a dish with some water over medium warmth, include asparagus, cook for 8 min, drain well, chop two spears, and save the rest.

2. Heat up a frying-pan with the oil over medium warmth, include garlic, chopped asparagus, and onions, mix and cook for 5 min.

3. Include eggs, salt, and pepper, mix, spread, and cook for 5 min.

4. Lay out the whole asparagus on top of your frittata, sprinkle feta, present in the grill at 350 degrees F, and heat for 9 min.

5. Serve onto plates. Relax and enjoy!

Nourishment: calories 340. Grams: fat 12, fiber 3, carbs 8, protein 26.

Uncommon Breakfast Eggs

Prep & Cooking time: 1 hour

Serves: 12

Ingredients:

- Four tea bags
- Four tablespoons salt
- 12 eggs
- Two tablespoons cinnamon
- 6-star anise

- One teaspoon black pepper
- One tablespoon peppercorns
- 8 cups of water
- 1 cup tamari sauce

Directions:

1. Pour water into a clean pot, include eggs, heat them to the point of boiling over medium warmth and cook until they are hard boiled.

2. Chill them off and peel them. Cut them in half.

3. In a large pot, blend water in with tea bags, salt, pepper, peppercorns, cinnamon, star anise, and tamari sauce.

4. Include hard-boiled eggs, stir the pot, bring to a stew over low warmth and cook for 30 min.

5. Dispose of tea bags and cook eggs for another 10 min.

6. Leave eggs to chill off, and serve them for breakfast.

Relax and enjoy!

Nourishment: calories 90. Grams: fat 6, fiber 0, carbs 0, protein 7.

Eggs Baked in Avocados

Prep & Cooking time: 30 minutes

Serves: 4

Ingredients:

- Two avocados, cut in equal parts and pitted
- Four eggs
- Salt and black pepper to taste
- One tablespoon chives, chopped

Directions:

1. Scoop out the avo from the avocado halves and organize them in a heating dish.

2. Break an egg in every avocado, garnish with salt and pepper, put them in the stove at 425 degrees F, and heat for 20 min.

3. Sprinkle chives toward the end and serve for breakfast!

Relax and enjoy!

Nourishment: calories 400. Grams: fat 34, fiber 13, carbs 13, protein 15.

Shrimp and Bacon Breakfast

Prep & Cooking time: 25 minutes
Serves: 4
Ingredients:

- 1 cup mushrooms, sliced
- Four bacon slices, chopped
- 4 ounces smoked salmon, sliced
- 4 ounces shrimp, deveined
- Salt and black pepper to taste
- ½ cup coconut cream

Directions:

1. Heat up a frying-pan over medium warmth, include bacon, mix and cook for 5 min.
2. Include mushrooms, mix, and cook for 5 min more.
3. Include salmon, mix, and cook for 3 min.
4. Include shrimp and cook for 2 min.
5. Add salt, pepper, and coconut cream, mix again, cook for a short time, take off warmth, and serve onto plates.

Nourishment: calories 340. Grams: fat 23, fiber 1, carbs 4, protein 17.

Delectable Mexican Breakfast

Prep & Cooking time: 40 minutes
Serves: 8
Ingredients:

- ½ cup enchilada sauce
- 1 pound pork, ground
- 1 pound chorizo, sliced
- Salt and black pepper to taste
- Eight eggs
- One tomato, sliced
- Three tablespoons ghee
- ½ cup red onion, sliced
- One avocado, de-stoned, peeled, and sliced

Directions:
1. In a bowl, blend pork in with chorizo, mix, and spread on a lined heating tray.
2. Spread enchilada sauce on top, put under the grill at 350 degrees F and prepare for 20 min.
3. Heat up a frying-pan with the ghee over medium warmth, include eggs, and scramble them well.
4. Remove pork blend from the grill and spread fried eggs over them.
5. Sprinkle salt, pepper, tomato, onion, avocado, put onto plates, and serve.
Relax and enjoy!
Nourishment: calories 400. Grams: fat 32, fiber 4, carbs 7, protein 25.

Flavorful Breakfast Pie

Prep & Cooking time: 55 minutes
Serves: 8
Ingredients:
- ½ onion chopped
- One pie crust
- ½ red bell pepper, sliced
- ¾ pound hamburger, ground
- Salt and black pepper to taste
- Three tablespoons taco sauce
- A modest bunch of cilantro, sliced
- Eight eggs
- One teaspoon coconut oil
- Mango salsa for serving

Directions:
1. Heat up a frying-pan with the oil over medium warmth, include hamburger, cook until it is brown, and blend in with salt, pepper, and taco sauce.
2. Mix once more, move to a bowl and leave aside for the time being.
3. Heat up the frying-pan again over medium warmth with cooking juices from the meat, include onion and bell pepper, mix and cook for 4 min.

4. Include eggs, some salt, and mix well.

5. Include cilantro, mix again, and take off warmth.

6. Spread hamburger blend in pie covering, include veggies blend and spread over the meat, place in the oven at 350 degrees F and prepare for 45 min.

7. Leave the pie to chill off a while, slice, put onto plates, and present with mango salsa on top.

Relax and enjoy!

Nourishment: calories 198. Grams: fat 11, fiber 1, carbs 12, protein 12

Breakfast Stir Fry

Prep & Cooking time: 40 minutes

Serves: 2

Ingredients:

- ½ pounds hamburger meat, minced
- Two teaspoons red bean stew drops
- One tablespoon tamari sauce
- Two bell peppers, chopped
- One teaspoon bean stew powder
- One tablespoon coconut oil
- Salt and black pepper to taste

For the bok choy:

- Six bundles bok choy, cleaned and chopped
- One teaspoon ginger, ground
- Salt to taste
- One tablespoon coconut oil

For the eggs:

- One tablespoon coconut oil
- Two eggs

Directions:

1. Heat up a frying-pan with one tablespoon of coconut oil over medium-high warmth, include hamburger and bell peppers, mix and cook for 10 min.

2. Place salt, pepper, tamari sauce, stew pieces, and stew powder, stir, cook for 4 min more and take off warmth.

3. Heat up another dish with one tablespoon oil over medium warmth, include bok choy, mix and cook for 3 min.

4. Place salt and ginger, mix, cook for 2 min more and take off warmth.

5. Heat up the third dish with one tablespoon oil over medium warmth, split eggs and fry them.

6. Separate hamburger and bell pepper blend into two dishes.

7. Separate bok choy and top with eggs.

Relax and enjoy!

Nourishment: calories 248, fat 14, fiber 4, carbs 10, protein 14

Breakfast Bar with Apple and Cinnamon

Prep & Cooking time: 40 minutes   (see conversion table on p. 127 for Imperial measures)Serves: 8

Ingredients:

- 4 eggs
- 150 g of ground pecan nuts
- 50 g coconut oil
- some freeze-dried apple pieces
- 2 teaspoons of cinnamon
- 1 teaspoon vanilla extract
- 10 drops of liquid Stevia (an artificial sweetener)

Directions

1. First preheat the oven to 180 ° C. Meanwhile, mix the eggs, coconut oil, vanilla extract, stevia, and cinnamon thoroughly.

2. Now add in the apples and nuts and mix everything vigorously.

3. Pour the dough into a baking dish, spread it evenly, and bake at a temperature of 180 ° C for about 25 minutes. Then divide into even bars and serve.

Almond Paste

Prep & Cooking time: 20 minutes
Serves:1
Ingredients:
- 200 ml of hot water
- 1 tbsp. coconut oil
- 10 g gold linseed
- 60 g ground almonds
- some xylitol (an artificial sweetener)
- Fruit as you like

Directions

1. Mix the almonds, the hot water, coconut oil, and xylitol in a vessel and puree to a fine mass using a hand blender.
2. Fill the finished porridge into a bowl and garnish with berries or other fruits.

Bacon & Egg

Prep & Cooking time: 30 minutes
Serves: 2
Ingredients:
- 1 large zucchini
- 4 slices of bacon
- 50 g parmesan cheese
- 4 eggs
- some salt and pepper

Directions

1. First cut the bacon into strips and fry some fat in a pan until crispy.
2. Then bring the zucchini into a noodle shape in a spiral cutter and put it on the stove. Season everything well.
3. Finely grate the parmesan. Use a spoon to form 4 wells in the zucchini noodles and add some parmesan to each. Also, insert one of the eggs in each case.

4. Simmer everything for a while and then cook covered again for 3 minutes until the zucchini base is crispy and the fried eggs are cooked.

Breakfast muffins

Prep & Cooking time: 25 minutes
Serves: 2
Ingredients:
- some olive oil
- 300 g spinach
- 4 eggs
- 100 g grated cheese
- 500 g of brown mushrooms
- 2 tbsp. whipped cream
- 12 slices of bacon
- some salt and pepper

Directions

1. Set the oven to a temperature of 180 ° C and let a dash of oil in the pan get hot during this time. First, clean the mushrooms, then add them to the pan and let them soften. Set the mushrooms aside for now.

2. Also heat the spinach in a pan and then add 40 ml of water. Now let the spinach simmer for a few minutes, but only long enough so that it doesn't collapse. Now drain the spinach thoroughly.

3. Mix all the eggs in a container and add the mushrooms, spinach, grated cheese, and cream. Mix everything and season well.

4. Grease 12 muffin tins and roll a slice of bacon into each one. Then fill up all the shapes with the egg mixture. Let everything cook for 25 minutes in the oven.

Cloud Bread

Prep & Cooking time: 40 minutes

Serves: 1

Ingredients:

- 100 g cream cheese
- 3 eggs
- a bit of salt
- ½ teaspoon baking powder

Directions

1. In the first step: separate the egg yolk and egg white and whip the egg white with a little salt to form a mixture. Also preheat the oven to 130 ° C.

2. In a separate bowl, mix the egg yolks with the baking powder and cream cheese and stir thoroughly.

3. Slowly fold the egg white mix into the egg yolk mixture. Place the resulting mixture on a baking sheet lined with baking paper. You should create 5 identical flat cakes. Bake them at 130 ° C for half an hour.

Lunch

Basic Asparagus Lunch

Prep & Cooking time: 20 minutes
Servings: 4
Ingredients:
- 2 egg yolks
- Salt and black pepper to taste
- ¼ cup ghee
- 1 tablespoon lemon juice
- A spot of cayenne pepper
- 40 asparagus spears

Directions:
1. In a bowl, whisk egg yolks thoroughly.
2. Move this to a little frying-pan over low warmth.
3. Add lemon squeeze and whisk well.
4. Add ghee and stir until it softens.
5. Add a pinch of salt, pepper, and cayenne pepper ,and whisk again well.
6. Then, heat a frying-pan over medium-high warmth, add asparagus spears, and fry them for 5 minutes.
7. Separate asparagus on plates, drizzle the sauce you've made on top, and serve.
Relax and enjoy!
Nourishment: calories 150. Grams: fat 13, fiber 6, carbs 2, protein 3.

Straightforward Shrimp Pasta

Prep & Cooking time: 10 minutes
Servings: 4
Ingredients:
- 12 ounces egg noodles
- 2 tablespoons olive oil
- Salt and black pepper to taste
- 2 tablespoons ghee

• 4 garlic cloves, minced
• 1 pound shrimp, crude, peeled and deveined
• Juice of ½ lemon
• ½ teaspoon paprika
• A small bunch of basil, chopped

Directions:

1. Place water in a pot, add some salt, heat to the point of boiling, add noodles, cook for 2 minutes, drain them, and move to a warmed dish.

2. Toast noodles for a couple of moments, take off warmth and leave them aside.

3. Heat up a dish with the ghee and olive oil over medium warmth, add garlic, mix, and brown for a few moments.

4. Add shrimp and lemon squeeze and cook for 3 minutes on each side.

5. Add noodles, salt, pepper, and paprika mix. Separate into bowls; furthermore, serve with sliced basil on top.

Relax and enjoy!

Nourishment: calories 300. Grams: fat 20, fiber 6, carbs 3, protein 30.

Staggering Mexican Meal

Prep & Cooking time: 45 minutes
Servings: 6
Ingredients:
• 2 chipotle peppers, chopped
• 2 jalapenos, chopped
• 1 tablespoon olive oil
• ¼ cup full cream
• 1 little white onion, chopped
• Salt and black pepper to taste
• 1 pound chicken thighs, skinless, boneless, and chopped
• 1 cup red enchilada sauce
• 4 ounces cream cheddar
• Cooking fat
• 1 cup pepper jack cheddar, grated

- 2 tablespoons cilantro (i.e. coriander), chopped
- 2 tortillas

Directions:

1. Heat up a dish with the oil over medium warmth, add chipotle and jalapeno peppers, mix and cook for a couple of moments.
2. Add onion, mix, and cook for 5 minutes.
3. Add cream cheddar and full cream and mix until cheddar liquefies.
4. Add chicken, salt, pepper, and enchilada sauce, mix well, and take off warmth.
5. Oil a heating dish with cooking fat, place tortillas on the base, spread chicken blend once finished, and sprinkle grated cheddar.
6. Spread with tin foil, present in the grill at 350 degrees F, and heat for 15 minutes.
7. Eliminate the tin foil and heat for 15 minutes more.
8. Sprinkle cilantro on top and serve.

Relax and enjoy!

Nourishment: calories 240. Grams: fat 12, fiber 5, carbs 5, protein 20

Tasty Asian Lunch Serving of Mixed Greens

Prep & Cooking time: 25 minutes

Servings: 4

Ingredients:

- 1 pound meat, ground/minced
- 1 tablespoon sriracha (hot Vietnamese sauce)
- 2 tablespoons coconut oil
- 2 garlic cloves, minced
- 10 ounces coleslaw blend
- 2 tablespoon sesame seed oil
- Salt and black pepper to taste
- 1 teaspoon apple juice vinegar
- 1 teaspoon sesame seeds
- 1 green onion tail, chopped

Directions:

1. Heat up a frying-pan with the oil over medium warmth, add garlic and brown for a few moments.

2. Add meat, mix, and cook for 10 minutes.

3. Add coleslaw blend, toss to cover, and cook for 1minute.

4. Add vinegar, sriracha, coconut oil, salt, and pepper, also mix, cook for 4 minutes more.

5. Add green onions and sesame seeds, toss to cover, separate into bowls, and serve for lunch.

Relax and enjoy!

Nourishment: calories 350. Grams: fat 23, fiber 6, carbs 3, protein 20.

Straightforward Buffalo Wings

Prep & Cooking time: 30 minutes
Servings: 2
Ingredients:
• 2 tablespoons ghee
• 6 chicken wings, cut in equal parts
• Salt and black pepper to taste
• A touch of garlic powder
• ½ cup hot sauce
• A touch of cayenne pepper
• ½ teaspoon sweet paprika
Directions:
1. In a bowl, blend chicken pieces with half of the hot sauce, salt also, pepper, and toss well to cover.

2. Arrange chicken pieces on a lined heating dish, put in the preheated oven, and cook for 8 minutes.

3. Flip chicken pieces and grill for 8 minutes more.

4. Heat up a dish with the ghee over medium warmth.

5. Add the remainder of the hot sauce, salt, pepper, cayenne, and paprika, mix and cook for two or three minutes.

6. Move grilled chicken pieces to a bowl, add ghee and hot sauce blend over them and toss to cover well.

7. Serve them immediately!

Relax and enjoy!

Nourishment: calories 500. Grams: fat 45, fiber 12, carbs 1, protein 45.

Astounding Bacon and Mushroom Sticks

Prep & Cooking time: 30 minutes
Servings: 6
Ingredients:
- 1 pound mushroom caps
- 6 bacon strips
- Salt and black pepper to taste
- ½ teaspoon sweet paprika
- Some sweet mesquite seasoning

Directions:
1. Season mushroom caps with salt, pepper, and paprika.
2. Lance a bacon strip on a toothpich.
3. Lance a mushroom cap and lay over bacon.
4. Repeat until you get a mushroom and bacon mesh.
5. Repeat with the remainder of the mushrooms and bacon strips.
6. Season with sweet mesquite, place all sticks on preheated tray, and grill over medium warmth, cook for 10 minutes, flip and cook for 10 minutes more.
7. Separate onto plates and serve for lunch with a side serving of mixed greens!
Relax and enjoy!
Nourishment: calories 110. Grams: fat 7, fiber 4, carbs 2, protein 10.

Basic Tomato Soup

Prep & Cooking time: 15 minutes
Servings: 4
Ingredients:
- 1 quart canned tomato soup
- 4 tablespoons ghee
- ¼ cup olive oil
- ¼ cup intensely hot sauce
- 2 tablespoons apple juice vinegar
- Salt and black pepper to taste
- 1 teaspoon oregano, dried
- 2 teaspoon turmeric, ground

• 8 bacon strips, cooked and sliced
• A modest bunch of green onions, chopped
• A modest bunch of basil leaves, chopped
Directions:
1. Put tomato soup in a pot and warm up over medium warmth.
2. Add olive oil, ghee, hot sauce, vinegar, salt, pepper, turmeric, oregano; mix, and stew for 5 minutes.
3. Take off warmth, separate soup into bowls, top with Bacon slices, basil, and green onions.
Relax and enjoy!
Nourishment: calories 400. Grams: fat 34, fiber 7, carbs 10, protein 12.

Bacon-Wrapped Frankfurters

Prep & Cooking time: 40 minutes
Servings: 4
Ingredients:
• 8 bacon strips
• 8 hotdog sausages
• 16 pepper jack cheddar cuts
• Salt and black pepper to taste
• A touch of garlic powder
• ½ teaspoon sweet paprika
• 1 touch of onion powder
Directions:
1. Heat up your stove, grill over medium warmth, add hotdogs, cook for a couple of moments on each side, move to a plate, and leave them aside for a couple of moments to chill off.
2. Make a cut in every Wiener sausage to make pockets, stuff each with two cheddar cuts, and season with salt, pepper, paprika, onion, and garlic powder.
3. Envelop each stuffed hotdog by a bacon strip, secure with toothpicks, place on a lined preparing sheet, put into the oven at 400 degrees F, and prepare for 15 minutes.
4. Serve hot for lunch!

Relax and enjoy!
Nourishment: calories 500. Grams: fat 37, fiber 2, carbs 4, protein 40.

Lunch Lobster Bisque

Prep & Cooking time: 1 hour 10 minutes
Servings: 4
Ingredients:
• 4 garlic cloves, minced
• 1 little red onion, chopped
• 24 ounces lobster, pre-cooked
• Salt and black pepper to taste
• ½ cup tomato paste
• 2 carrots, finely chopped
• 4 celery stems, chopped
• 1-quart seafood stock
• 1 tablespoon olive oil
• 1 cup weighty cream
• 3 cloves
• 1 teaspoon thyme, dried
• 1 teaspoon peppercorns
• 1 teaspoon paprika
• 1 teaspoon thickener
• A modest bunch of parsley chopped
• 1 tablespoon lemon juice

Directions:
1. Heat up a pot with the oil over medium warmth, add onion, also mix, cook for 4 minutes.
2. Add garlic, mix, and cook for a short time more.
3. Add celery and carrot, mix and cook for a moment.
4. Add tomato paste and stock and mix everything.
5. Add cloves salt, pepper, peppercorns, paprika, thyme, thickener, mix, and stew over medium warmth for 60 minutes.
6. Dispose of cloves, add cream, and bring to a stew.
7. Mix utilizing a submersion blender, add lobster pieces and cook for a couple of moments more.

8. Add lemon juice, mix, separate into bowls, and sprinkle parsley on top.

Relax and enjoy!

Nourishment: calories 200. Grams: fat 12, fiber 7, carbs 6, protein 12.

Straightforward Halloumi Serving of Mixed Greens

Prep & Cooking time: 20 minutes
Servings: 1
Ingredients:
• 3 ounces halloumi or cheddar, cut
• 1 cucumber, cut
• 1-ounce pecans, chopped
• A shower of olive oil
• A small bunch of baby rocket/rucola
• 5 cherry tomatoes, split
• A sprinkle of balsamic vinegar
• Salt and black pepper to taste
Directions:
1. Heat up your grill over medium-high warmth, add halloumi pieces, barbecue them for 5 minutes on each side and move to a plate.
2. In a bowl, blend tomatoes with cucumber, pecans, and rucula/rocket.
3. Add halloumi pieces on top, season everything with salt, pepper, sprinkle the oil and the vinegar, toss to cover, and serve.

Relax and enjoy!

Nourishment: calories 450. Grams: fat 43, fiber 5, carbs 4, protein 21.

Delectable Mexican Lunch

Prep & Cooking time: 30 minutes
Serves: 4
Ingredients:
• ¼ cup cilantro/coriander, sliced
• Two avocados, de-stoned, peeled, and cut into pieces
• One tablespoon lime juice
• ¼ cup white onion, sliced

- One teaspoon garlic, minced
- Salt and black pepper to taste
- Six cherry tomatoes cut in quarters
- ½ cup of water
- 2-pound hamburger meat, ground
- 2 cups sour cream
- ¼ cup taco preparation
- 2 cups lettuce leaves, grated
- Some cayenne pepper sauce for serving
- 2 cups cheddar, grated

Directions:

1. In a bowl, blend cilantro with lime juice, avocado, onion, tomatoes, salt, pepper, and garlic, mix well and leave aside in the cooler until later.
2. Heat up a container over medium warmth, include meat, mix, and brown for 10 min.
3. Include taco preparation and water, mix and cook over medium-low warmth for 10 min. more.
4. Separate this blend into fourl bowls.
5. Include cream, avocado blend you've made before, lettuce pieces, and cheddar.
6. Sprinkle cayenne pepper sauce toward the end and serve for lunch! Relax and enjoy!

Nourishment: calories 340. Grams: fat 30, fiber 5, carbs 3, protein 32

Lunch Stuffed Peppers

Prep & Cooking time: 50 minutes
Serves: 4
Ingredients:
- Four sweet peppers with the stalk cut off, seeds eliminated and cut into equal parts the long way
- One tablespoon ghee
- Salt and black pepper to taste
- ½ teaspoon spices/herbs de Provence

- 1 pound sweet frankfurter, sliced
- Three tablespoons yellow onions, sliced
- Some marinara sauce
- A sprinkle of olive oil

Directions:

1. Sprinkle sweet peppers with salt and pepper, sprinkle the oil, rub well and prepare in the stove at 350 degrees F for 20 min.

2. In the interim, heat a frying-pan over medium warmth, include hotdog pieces, mix and cook for 5 min.

3. Include onion, herbs de Provence, salt, pepper, and ghee, mix well, and cook for 5 min.

4. Remove peppers from the grill, fill them with the hotdog blend, place them in an oven dish, sprinkle marinara sauce over them, put into the oven again, and heat for 10 min more.

5. Serve hot.

Relax and enjoy!

Nourishment: calories 320. Grams: fat 8, fiber 4, carbs 3, protein 10

Uncommon Lunch Burgers

Prep & Cooking time: 35 minutes
Serves: 8
Ingredients:

- 1 pound brisket, ground
- 1 pound hamburger, ground
- Salt and black pepper to taste
- Eight cheese slices
- One tablespoon garlic, minced
- One tablespoon Italian flavoring
- Two tablespoons mayonnaise
- One tablespoon ghee
- Two tablespoons olive oil
- One yellow onion, sliced
- One tablespoon water

Directions:

1. In a bowl, blend brisket with hamburger, salt, pepper, Italian flavoring, garlic, and mayo and mix well.

2. Shape eight patties and make a pocket in each.

3. Stuff every burger with a cheese slice and seal.

4. Heat up a container with the olive oil over medium warmth, include onions, mix and cook for 2 min.

5. Include the water, mix, and accumulate them toward the edge of the container.

6. Place burgers in the container with the onions and cook them over medium-low warmth for 10 min.

7. Flip them, include the ghee, and cook them for 10 min more.

8. Put burgers on buns and serve them with caramelized onions on top.

Nourishment: calories 180. Grams: fat 8, fiber 1, carbs 4, protein 20

Distinctive Burger

Prep & Cooking time: 40 minutes
Serves: 4
Ingredients:
 For the sauce:
- Four chili peppers, sliced
- 1 cup of water
- 1 cup almond spread
- One teaspoon turmeric
- Six tablespoons coconut oil
- Four garlic cloves, minced
- One tablespoon rice vinegar

For the burgers:
- Four pepper jack Cheddar slices
- One and a half pounds of meat, ground
- One red onion, sliced
- Eight bacon slices
- Eight lettuce leaves
- Salt and black pepper to taste

Directions:

1. Heat up a dish with the almond margarine over medium warmth.

2. Include water, mix well, and bring to a stew.

3. Include coconut oil and mix well.

4. In your food processor, blend bean stew peppers with garlic, turmeric, vinegar, and mix well.

5. Add this to almond margarine blend, mix well, take off warmth, and leave aside for the present.

6. In a bowl, blend meat in with salt and pepper, mix and shape four patties.

7. Place them in a dish, put in your preheated oven, and grill for 7 min.

8. Flip burgers and grill them for 7 min more.

9. Put cheddar slices on burgers, present in your oven, and grill for 4 min more.

10. Heat up a dish over medium warmth, include bacon slices and fry them for two or three min.

11. Put 2 lettuce leaves on a dish, include one burger top, at that point 1 onion slice and one bacon slice and top with some almond spread sauce.

12. Repeat with the remainder of the lettuce leaves, burgers, onion, bacon, and sauce.

Relax and enjoy!

Nourishment: calories 700. Grams: fat 56, fiber 10, carbs 7, protein 40

Delightful Zucchini Dish

Prep & Cooking time: 10 minutes
Serves: 1
Ingredients:

- One tablespoon olive oil
- Three tablespoons ghee
- 2 cups zucchini, cut with a spiralizer
- One teaspoon red pepper chips
- One tablespoon garlic, minced
- One tablespoon red bell pepper, sliced
- Salt and black pepper to taste

- One tablespoon basil, sliced
- ¼ cup asiago cheddar, sliced
- ¼ cup parmesan, ground

Directions:

1. Heat up a dish with the oil and ghee over medium warmth, include garlic, bell pepper, and pepper chips, mix and cook for a few moments.

2. Include zucchini noodles, mix, and cook for 2 min. more.

3. Include basil, parmesan, salt, and pepper, mix and cook for a couple of moments more.

4. Take off warmth, move to a bowl, and serve lunch with asiago cheddar on top.

Relax and enjoy!

Nourishment: calories 140. Grams: fat 3, fiber 1, carbs 1.3, protein 5

Bacon and Zucchini Noodles Salad

Prep & Cooking time: 10 minutes

Serves: 2

Ingredients:

- 1 cup baby spinach
- 4 cups zucchini noodles
- 1/3 cup bleu cheddar, sliced
- 1/3 cup thick cheddar dressing
- ½ cup bacon, cooked and sliced
- black pepper to taste

Directions:

1. In a plate of mixed greens bowl, blend spinach in with zucchini noodles, bacon, and bleu cheddar and toss.

2. Include cheddar dressing and black pepper to taste, toss well to cover, separate into two dishes, and serve.

Relax and enjoy!

Nourishment: calories 200, Grams: fat 14, fiber 4, carbs 2, protein 10

Astounding Chicken Salad

Prep & Cooking time: 10 minutes
Serves: 3
Ingredients:

- One green onion, sliced
- One celery rib, sliced
- One egg, hard-boiled, peeled and sliced
- 5 ounces chicken breast, cooked and sliced
- Two tablespoons parsley, sliced
- ½ tablespoons dill relish
- Salt and black pepper to taste
- 1/3 cup mayonnaise
- A spot of granulated garlic
- One teaspoon mustard

Directions:

1. In your food processor, blend parsley in with onion and celery and mix well.
2. Move these to a bowl and leave them aside for the present.
3. Put chicken meat in your food processor, mix well, and add to the veggies bowl.
4. Include egg pieces, salt and pepper, and mix.
5. Additionally, include mustard, mayo, dill relish, and granulated garlic, toss to cover, and serve immediately.

Relax and enjoy!
Nourishment: calories 283, Grams: fat 23, fiber 5, carbs 3, protein 12

Mind-Blowing Steak Salad

Prep & Cooking time: 30 minutes
Serves: 4
Ingredients:

- One and ½ pound steak, daintily sliced
- Three tablespoons avocado oil
- Salt and black pepper to taste
- ¼ cup balsamic vinegar

- 6 ounces sweet onion, sliced
- One lettuce head, sliced
- Two garlic cloves, minced
- 4 ounces mushrooms, sliced
- One avocado, de-stoned, peeled, and sliced
- 3 ounces sun-dried tomatoes, sliced
- One yellow bell pepper, sliced
- One orange bell pepper, sliced
- One teaspoon Italian flavoring
- One teaspoon red pepper chips
- One teaspoon onion powder

Directions:

1. In a bowl, blend steak pieces with some salt, pepper, and balsamic vinegar, toss to cover and leave to the side until later.

2. Heat up a frying-pan with the avocado oil over medium-low warmth, include mushrooms, garlic, salt, pepper, and onion, mix and cook for 20 min.

3. In a bowl, blend lettuce leaves with orange and yellow bell pepper, sun-dried tomatoes, and avocado and mix.

4. Sprinkle steak pieces with onion powder, pepper drops, and Italian flavoring.

5. Put steak pieces in a hot frying-pan, present in the preheated oven, and cook for 5 min.

6. Separate steak pieces on plates, include lettuce and avocado plateful of mixed greens on the side and top everything with onion and mushroom blend.

Relax and enjoy!

Nourishment: calories 435, Grams: fat 23, fiber 7, carbs 10, protein 35

Fennel and Chicken Lunch Salad

Prep & Cooking time: 10 minutes
Serves: 4
Ingredients:

- Three chicken breasts, boneless, skinless, cooked and sliced
- Two tablespoons pecan oil

- ¼ cup pecans, toasted and sliced
- One and ½ cup fennel, sliced
- Two tablespoons lemon juice
- ¼ cup mayonnaise
- Two tablespoons fennel fronds, sliced
- Salt and black pepper to taste

A spot of cayenne pepper

Directions:

1. In a bowl, blend fennel with chicken and pecans and mix.

2. In another bowl, blend mayo with salt, pepper, fennel fronds, pecan oil, lemon juice, cayenne, and garlic and mix well.

3. Pour this over chicken and fennel blend, toss to cover well, and keep in the cooler until you serve.

Relax and enjoy!

Nourishment: calories 200, Grams: fat 10, fiber 1, carbs 3, protein 7

Simple Stuffed Avocado

Prep & Cooking time: 10 minutes

Serves: 1

Ingredients:

- One avocado
- 4 ounces canned sardines, drained
- One spring onion, sliced
- One tablespoon mayonnaise
- One tablespoon lemon juice
- Salt and black pepper to taste
- ¼ teaspoon turmeric powder

Directions:

1. Cut avocado in equal parts, take out the pip, and put in a bowl.

2. Mash with a fork and blend in with sardines.

3. Mash again with your fork and blend in with the onion, lemon juice, turmeric powder, salt, pepper, and mayo.

4. Mix everything and separate it into avocado halves.

5. Serve for lunch immediately.

Relax and enjoy!
Nourishment: calories 230, Grams: fat 34, fiber 12, carbs 5, protein 27

Pesto Chicken Salad

Prep & Cooking time: 10 minutes
Serves: 4
Ingredients:
- 1 pound chicken meat, cooked and cubed
- Salt and black pepper to taste
- Ten cherry tomatoes, divided
- Six bacon slices, cooked and sliced
- ¼ cup mayonnaise
- One avocado, de-stoned, peeled, and cubed
- Two tablespoons garlic pesto

Directions:
1. In a salad bowl, blend chicken in with bacon, avocado, tomatoes, salt and pepper, and mix.
2. Include mayo and garlic pesto, toss well to cover, and serve.
Relax and enjoy!
Nourishment: calories 357, Grams: fat 23, fiber 5, carbs 3, protein 26

Scrumptious Lunch Salad

Prep & Cooking time: 20 minutes
Serves: 1
Ingredients:
- 4 ounces hamburger steak
- 2 cups lettuce leaves, grated
- Salt and black pepper to taste
- Cooking oil
- Two tablespoons cilantro, sliced
- Two radishes, sliced
- 1/3 cup red cabbage, grated
- Three tablespoons shaken chimichurri sauce

- One tablespoons salad dressing
  For the plate of salad dressing:
- Three garlic cloves, minced
- ½ teaspoon Worcestershire sauce
- One tablespoon mustard
- ½ cup apple juice vinegar
- ¼ cup of water
- ½ cup olive oil
- ¼ teaspoon Tabasco sauce
- Salt and black pepper to taste

Directions:

1. In a bowl, blend garlic cloves in Worcestershire sauce, mustard, juice vinegar, water, olive oil, salt, pepper, and Tabasco sauce, whisk well and leave aside until later.

2. Heat up your stove grill over medium-high warmth, shower cooking oil, include steak, sprinkle with salt and pepper, cook for 4 min, flip, cook for 4 min more, take off warmth, leave aside to chill off and cut into slim strips.

3. In a salad bowl, blend lettuce in with cilantro, cabbage, radishes, chimichurri sauce, and steak strips.

4. Include one tablespoon of the salad dressing, toss to cover, and serve immediately.

Relax and enjoy!

Nourishment: calories 456, Grams: fat 32, fiber 2, carbs 6, protein 30

Simple Lunch Crab Cakes

Prep & Cooking time: 25 minutes
Serves: 6
Ingredients:

- 1 pound crabmeat
- ¼ cup parsley, sliced
- Salt and black pepper to taste
- Two green onions, sliced
- ¼ cup cilantro, sliced
- One teaspoon jalapeno pepper, minced
- One teaspoon lemon juice
- One teaspoon Worcestershire sauce
- One teaspoon clove flavoring
- ½ teaspoon mustard powder
- ½ cup mayonnaise
- One egg
- Two tablespoons olive oil

Directions:

1. In a big bowl, blends crab meat with salt, pepper, parsley, green onions, cilantro, jalapeno, lemon juice, clove flavoring, mustard powder, and Worcestershire sauce and mix well overall.

2. In another bowl, blend egg, mind mayo, and whisk.

3. Add this to the crabmeat blend and mix everything.

4. Shape six patties from this blend and put them on a plate.

5. Heat up a frying-pan with the oil over medium-high warmth, include three crab cakes, cook for 3 min, flip, cook them for 3 min more, and move to paper towels.

6. Repeat with the other three crab cakes, drain excess oil, and serve for lunch.

Relax and enjoy!

Nourishment: calories 254, Grams: fat 17, fiber 1, carbs 1, protein 20

Dinner

Paprika Chicken

Prep & Cooking Time: 35 minutes
Servings: 4
Ingredients:

- 2 Teaspoons Smoked Paprika
- ½ Cup Full-Fat Whipping Cream
- ½ Cup Sweet Onion, Chopped
- 1 Tablespoon Olive Oil
- 4 Chicken Breasts, Skin on & 4 Ounces Each
- ½ Cup Sour Cream
- 2 Tablespoons Parsley, Chopped

Directions:

1. Season your chicken with salt and pepper, putting a frying-pan over medium-high heat. Add your oil, and once it simmers, grill your chicken on both sides. It should take about fifteen minutes to cook your chicken all the way through. Put your chicken to the side.
2. Add in your onion, sautéing for four minutes, or until tender.
3. Stir in your paprika and cream, bringing it to a simmer.
4. Return your chicken to the frying-pan, simmering for five more minutes.
5. Stir in sour cream and serve topped with parsley.

Nutrition: Calories: 389 Grams Protein: 25 Grams Fat: 30 Grams Net Carbs: 4 Grams.

Coconut Chicken

Prep & Cooking Time: 40 minutes
Servings: 4
Ingredients:

- 1 Teaspoon Ground Cumin
- 1 Teaspoon Ground Coriander
- ¼ Cup Cilantro, Fresh & Chopped

- 1 Cup of Coconut Milk
- 1 Tablespoon Curry Powder
- ½ Cup Sweet Onion, Chopped
- 2 Tablespoons Olive Oil
- 4 Chicken Breasts, 4 Ounces Each & Cut Into 2 Inch Chunks

Directions:

1. Use a saucepan, adding in your oil, and heating it over medium-high heat.
2. Sauté your chicken until it's almost completely cooked, which will take roughly ten minutes.
3. Add in your onion, cooking for another three minutes.
4. Whisk your curry powder, coconut milk, coriander, and cumin together.
5. Pour the sauce into your pan, bringing it to a boil with your chicken.
6. Reduce the heat, and let it simmer for ten minutes.
7. Serve topped with cilantro.

Nutrition: Calories: 382 Protein: 23 Grams Fat: 31 Grams Net Carbs: 4 Grams

Cabbage & Chicken Plate

Prep & Cooking Time: 25 minutes
Servings: 4
Ingredients:

- 1 Cup Bean Sprouts, Fresh
- 2 Tablespoons Sesame & Garlic Flavored Oil
- ½ Cup Onion, Sliced
- 4 Cups Bok Choy, Shredded
- 3 Stalks Celery, Chopped
- 1 Tablespoon Ginger, Minced
- 2 Tablespoon Coconut Oil
- 1 Teaspoon Stevia
- 1 Cup Chicken Broth
- 1 ½ Teaspoons Minced Garlic
- 1 Teaspoon Arrowroot

- 4 Chicken Breasts, Boneless, Cooked & Sliced Thin

Directions:

1. Shred your cabbage, and then add your chicken and onion together.
2. Add in a dollop of mayonnaise if desired, drizzling with oil.
3. Season as desired and serve.

Nutrition: Calories: 368 Grams Protein: 42 Grams Fat: 18 Grams Net Carbs: 8 Grams.

Grilled Chicken & Cheesy Spinach

Prep & Cooking Time: 20 minutes
Servings: 6
Ingredients:

- 3 Ounces Mozzarella Cheese
- 3 Chicken Breasts, Large & Sliced in Half
- 10 Ounces Spinach, Frozen, Thawed & Drained
- ½ Cup Roasted Red Peppers, Sliced Into Strips
- 2 Cloves Minced Garlic
- 1 Teaspoon Olive Oil
- Sea Salt & Black Pepper to Taste

Directions:

1. Start by heating your oven to 400 deg. F, and then grease a pan.
2. Bake your chicken breasts for two to three minutes per side.
3. In a frying-pan, cook your garlic and spinach in oil for three minutes.
4. Put your chicken in a pan, topping it with spinach, roasted peppers and mozzarella.
5. Bake until your cheese melts - and serve warm.

Nutrition: Calories: 195 Grams Protein: 30 Grams Fat: 7 Grams Net Carbs: 3 Grams.

Balsamic Chicken with Vegetables

Prep & Cooking Time: 40 minutes
Servings: 4
Ingredients:

- 8 Chicken Cutlets, Skinless & Boneless
- ½ Cup Buttermilk
- 4 Tablespoons Dijon Mustard
- 2/3 Cup Almond Meal
- 2/3 Cup Chopped Cashews
- 4 Teaspoons Stevia
- ¾ Teaspoon Rosemary
- Sea Salt & Black Pepper to Taste

Directions:

1. Start by heating your oven to 425 deg. F.
2. Mix your buttermilk and mustard in a bowl.
3. Add your chicken, coating it.
4. Put a frying-pan over medium heat, and then add in your almond meal. Bake until it's golden, putting it in a bowl.
5. Add your sea salt, pepper, rosemary, and cashews, mixing well. Coat your chicken with the almond meal mix, and then put it in a baking pan.
6. Bake for twenty-five minutes.

Nutrition: Calories: 248 Grams Protein: 27 Grams Fat: 8 Grams Net Carbs: 14 Grams.

Steak & Broccoli Medley

Prep & Cooking Time: 20 minutes
Servings: 4
Ingredients:

- 4 Ounces Butter
- ¾ lb. Ribeye Steak
- 9 Ounces Broccoli
- 1 Yellow Onion
- 1 Tablespoon Coconut Oil
- 1 Tablespoon Pumpkin Seeds

- Sea Salt & Black Pepper as Needed

Directions:

1. Slice your onion and steak before chopping your broccoli.
2. Put a frying pan over medium heat, adding in butter. Let it melt, and then add meat. Season with salt and pepper, placing your meat to the side.
3. Brown your onion and broccoli, adding more butter as necessary.
4. Add in your coconut oil before adding your meat back.
5. Serve topped with pumpkin seeds and butter.

Nutrition: Calories: 875 Grams Protein: 40 Grams Fat: 75 Grams Net Carbs: 10 Grams.

Stuffed Meat Loaf

Prep & Cooking Time: 1 hour 20 minutes
Servings: 8
Ingredients:

- 17 Ounces Ground Beef
- ¼ Cup Onions, Diced
- 6 Slices Cheddar Cheese
- ¼ Cup Green Onions, Diced
- ½ Cup Spinach
- ¼ Cup Mushrooms

Directions:

1. Mix your salt, pepper, meat, cumin, and garlic before greasing a pan.
2. Put your cheese on the bottom of your meatloaf, adding in the spinach, mushrooms, and onions, and then use leftover meat to cover the top.
3. Bake at 350 deg. F for an hour, before serving.

Nutrition: Calories: 248 Grams Protein: 15 Grams Fat: 20 Grams Net Carbs: 1 Gram.

Beef Cabbage Rolls

Prep & Cooking Time: 6 hours 30 minutes
Servings: 5
Ingredients:

- 3 ½ lb. Corned Beef
- 15 Cabbage Leaves, Large
- 1 Onion
- 1 Lemon
- ¼ Cup Coffee
- ¼ Cup White Wine
- 1 Tablespoon Bacon Fat, Rendered
- 1 Tablespoon Brown Mustard
- 2 Tablespoons Himalayan Pink Sea Salt
- 2 Tablespoons Worcestershire Sauce
- 1 Teaspoon Whole Peppercorns
- 1 Teaspoon Mustard Seeds
- ½ Teaspoon Red Pepper Flakes
- ¼ Teaspoons Cloves
- ¼ Teaspoon Allspice
- 1 Bay Leaf, Large

Directions:

1. Add your liquids, corned beef, and spices into a slow cooker, cooking on low for six hours.
2. Bring a pot of water to a boil, adding your cabbage leaves and one sliced onion, bringing it to a boil for three minutes.
3. Remove your cabbage, putting it in ice water for three to four minutes, continuing to boil your onion.
4. Dry the leaves off, slicing your meat, and adding in your cooked onion and meat into your leaves.

Nutrition: Calories: 481 Grams Protein: 35 Grams Fat: 25 Grams Net Carbs: 4 Grams.

Zucchini Fettuccine with Beef

Prep & Cooking Time: 45 minutes
Servings: 4
Ingredients:

- 15 oz. ground beef
- 3 tbsp.. butter
- 1 yellow onion
- 8 oz. mushrooms
- 1 tbsp.. dried thyme
- ½ tsp.. salt
- 1 pinch ground black pepper
- 8 oz. blue cheese
- 1½ cups sour cream

Zucchini fettuccine:

- 2 zucchinis
- 1 oz. olive oil or butter
- Salt and pepper

Directions:

1. Peel the onion and chop it finely.
2. Melt the butter and sauté the onion until the onions are softened and transparent.
3. Add the ground beef and fry this for a few more minutes with the onion until it is browned and cooked through.
4. Slice or dice the mushrooms, and add them to the ground beef. Sauté the mushrooms with the beef mixture for a few minutes more, or until lightly brown.
5. Season it with thyme, salt, and pepper. Crumble the cheese over the hot mixture. Stir it well.
6. Add the sour cream and bring the mixture to a light boil. Lower the heat to a medium-low setting and let it simmer for about 10 minutes.

Zucchini fettuccine:

1. Calculate about one medium-sized zucchini per person.
2. Slice the zucchini lengthwise in half.

3. Scoop out the seeds with a spoon and slice the halves super thinly, lengthwise (julienne) with a potato peeler, or you can use a spiralizer to make zoodles (zucchini noodles.)
4. Toss the zucchini in some hot sauce of your choice, and serve it immediately.
5. If you are not going to be serving your zucchini with a hot sauce, then boil half a gallon of salted water in a large pot and parboil the zucchini slices for a minute. This makes it easier to eat.
6. Drain the water from the pot and add some olive oil or a knob of butter. Salt and pepper to taste.

Nutrition: Calories: 456 Grams Protein: 32 Grams Fat: 15 Grams Net Carbs: 13 Grams.

Oven-Baked Chicken in Garlic Butter

Prep & Cooking Time:1 hour 55 minutes
Servings: 3
Ingredients:
- 3 lbs. chicken, a whole bird
- 2 tsp. sea salt
- ½ tsp. ground black pepper
- 51/3 oz. butter
- 2 garlic cloves, minced

Directions:
1. Preheat the oven to 400°F.
2. Season the chicken with salt and pepper, both inside and out.
3. The chicken must go breast-side-up in the baking dish.
4. Combine the garlic and butter in a saucepan over medium heat. The butter should not turn brown or burn, just melt it gently.
5. Let the butter cool down once it is melted.
6. Pour the garlic butter mixture all over and inside the chicken. Bake the chicken on the lower oven rack for 1 to1 ½ hours, or until the internal temperature reaches 180°F. Baste it with the juices from the bottom of the pan every 20 minutes.
7. Serve with the juices.

Nutrition: Calories: 148 Grams Protein: 39 Grams Fat: 24 Grams Net Carbs: 16 Grams.

Keto Buffalo Drumsticks and Chili Aioli

Prep & Cooking Time: 55 minutes
Servings: 6
Ingredients:

- 2 lbs. chicken drumsticks or chicken wings
- 2 tbsp.. olive oil or coconut oil
- 2 tbsp.. white wine vinegar
- 1 tbsp.. tomato paste
- 1 tsp. salt
- 1 tsp. paprika powder
- 1 tablespoon Tabasco
- Butter or olive oil, for greasing the baking dish

Chili aioli:

- 2/3 cup mayonnaise
- 1 tablespoon smoked paprika powder or smoked chili powder
- 1 garlic clove, minced

Directions:

1. Preheat the oven to 450°F (220°C).
2. Put the drumsticks in a plastic bag.
3. Mix the ingredients for the marinade and pour them into the plastic bag. Shake the bag and let eveything marinate for 10 minutes.
4. Coat a baking dish with oil. Place the drumsticks in the baking bowl and let them bake for 30–40 minutes, or until they are done and have turned a beautiful color.
5. Mix mayonnaise, garlic, and chili, to serve with the drumsticks.

Nutrition: Calories: 409 Grams Protein: 22 Grams Fat: 10 Grams Net Carbs: 6 Grams.

Keto Fish Casserole

Prep & Cooking Time: 30 minutes
Servings: 4
Ingredients:

- 2 tbsp. olive oil
- 15 oz. broccoli
- 6 scallions
- 2 tbsp. small capers
- 1/6 oz. butter, for greasing the casserole dish
- 25 oz. white fish, in serving-sized pieces
- 1¼ cups full-fat whipping cream
- 1 tbsp. Dijon mustard
- 1 tsp. salt
- ¼ tsp. ground black pepper
- 1 tbsp. dried parsley
- 3 oz. butter

Directions:

1. Preheat the oven to 400°F.
2. Divide the broccoli into smaller floret heads and include the stems. Peel it with a sharp knife or a potato peeler if the stem is rough or leafy.
3. Fry the broccoli florets in oil on medium-high heat for about 5 minutes, until they are golden and soft. Season with salt and pepper to taste.
4. Add finely chopped scallions and the capers. Fry this for another 1 to 2 minutes and place the vegetables in a baking dish that has been greased.
5. Place the fish tightly in amongst the vegetables.
6. Mix the parsley, whipping cream, and mustard together. Pour this over the fish and vegetables. Top it with slices of butter.
7. Bake the fish until it is cooked through, and it flakes easily with a fork. Serve as is, or with a tasty green salad.

Nutrition: Calories: 314 Grams Protein: 20 Grams Fat: 8 Grams Net Carbs: 5 Grams.

Slow Cooker Keto Pork Roast

Prep & Cooking Time: 8 hours 55 minutes
Servings: 4
Ingredients:

- 30 oz. pork shoulder or pork roast
- ½ tbsp. salt
- 1 bay leaf
- 5 black peppercorns
- 2½ cups water
- 2 tsp. dried thyme or dried rosemary
- 2 garlic cloves
- 1½ oz. fresh ginger
- 1 tbsp. olive oil or coconut oil
- 1 tbsp. paprika powder
- ½ tsp. ground black pepper

Creamy gravy:

- 1½ cups full-fat whipping cream
- Juices from the roast

Directions:

1. Preheat the oven to a low heat of 200°F.
2. Season the meat with salt and place it into a deep baking dish.
3. Add water. Add a bay leaf, peppercorns, and thyme for more seasoning. Place the baking bowl in the oven for 7 to 8 hours and cover it with aluminum foil.
4. If you are using a slow cooker for this, do the same process as in step 2, only add 1 cup of water. Cook it for 8 hours on low or for 4 hours on high setting.
5. Take the meat out of the baking dish, and keep the pan juices in a separate pan to make gravy.
6. Turn the oven up to 450°F.
7. Finely chop or press the garlic and ginger into a small bowl. Add the oil, herbs, and pepper, and stir well to combine.
8. Rub the meat with the garlic and herb mixture.

9. Return the meat to the baking dish, and roast it for about 10 to 15 minutes or until it looks golden-brown.
10. Cut the meat into thin slices to serve it with the creamy gravy and a fiber-rich vegetable side dish.

Gravy:
1. Strain the reserved pan juices to get rid of any solid pieces from the liquid. Boil and reduce the pan juices to about half the original volume, this should be about 1 cup.
2. Pour the reduction into a pot with the whipping cream. Bring this to a boil. Reduce the heat and let it simmer to your desired consistency for a creamy gravy.

Nutrition: Calories: 432 Grams Protein: 15 Grams Fat: 29 Grams Net Carbs: 13 Grams.

Fried Eggs with Kale and Pork

Prep & Cooking Time: 35 minutes
Servings: 5
Ingredients:
- ½ lb kale
- 3 oz. butter
- 6 oz. smoked pork belly or bacon
- ¼ cup frozen cranberries
- 1 oz. pecans or walnuts
- 4 eggs
- Salt and pepper

Directions:
1. Cut and chop the kale into large squares. You can use pre-washed baby kale as a shortcut if you want. Melt two-thirds of the butter in a frying pan, and fry the kale on high heat until it is lightly browned around its edges.
2. Remove the kale from the frying pan and put it aside. Grill the pork belly in the same frying pan until it is crispy.
3. Turn the heat down. Put the sautéed kale back into the pan and add the cranberries and nuts. Stir this mixture until it is warmed through. Put it into a bowl on the side.

4. Turn up the heat once more, and fry the eggs in the remaining amount of the butter. Add salt and pepper to taste. Serve the eggs and greens immediately.

Nutrition: Calories: 180 Grams Protein: 23 Grams Fat: 30 Grams Net Carbs: 13 Grams.

Chicken Meatloaf

Prep & Cooking time: 50 minutes
Servings: 8
Ingredients:
• 1 cup Keto marinara sauce
• 2 pounds of chicken meat, ground/minced
• 2 tablespoons parsley, chopped
• 4 garlic cloves, minced
• 2 teaspoons onion powder
• 2 teaspoons Italian flavoring
• Salt and black pepper to taste
• For the filling:
• ½ cup ricotta cheddar
• 1 cup parmesan, ground
• 1 cup mozzarella, grated
• 2 teaspoons chives, chopped
• 2 tablespoons parsley, chopped
• 1 garlic clove, minced.

Directions:
1. In a bowl, blend chicken with half of the marinara sauce, salt, pepper, Italian flavoring, four garlic cloves, onion powder, and two tablespoons parsley; and mix well.
2. In another bowl, blend ricotta with half of the parmesan, half of the mozzarella, chives, one garlic clove, salt, pepper, and two tablespoons of parsley. Mix well.
3. Put half of the chicken blend into a portion container and spread equally.
4. Add cheddar filling and spread.
5. Top with the remainder of the meat and spread once more.

6. Put meatloaf in the stove at 400 degrees F and cook for 20 minutes.

7. Remove meatloaf from the stove, spread the remainder of the marinara sauce, the remainder of the parmesan, and mozzarella, and cook for 20 minutes more.

8. Leave meatloaf to chill off, cut, separateserve onto plates, and serve.

Relax and enjoy!

Nourishment: calories 273, Grams: fat 14, fiber 1, carbs 4, protein 28.

Delectable Entire Chicken

Prep & Cooking time: 50 minutes
Servings: 12
Ingredients:
• 1 entire chicken
• ½ teaspoon onion powder
• ½ teaspoon garlic powder
• Salt and black pepper to taste
• 2 tablespoons coconut oil
• 1 teaspoon Italian flavoring
• 1 and ½ cups chicken stock
• 2 teaspoons guar gum
Directions:
1. Rub chicken with half of the oil, garlic powder, salt, pepper, Italian flavoring, and onion powder.
2. Put the remainder of the oil into a pot and add chicken to it.
3. Add stock, stir pot, and cook on High for 40 minutes.
4. Move chicken to a platter and leave aside until later.
5. Set the pot on Sauté mode, add guar gum, mix and cook until it thickens.
6. Pour sauce over chicken and serve.

Relax and enjoy!

Nourishment: calories 450, Grams fat 30, fiber 1, carbs 1, protein 34.

Chicken and Green Onion Sauce

Prep & Cooking time: 40 minutes
Servings: 4
Ingredients:
• 2 tablespoons ghee
• 1 green onion, sliced
• 4 chicken breast parts, skinless and boneless
• Salt and black pepper to taste
• 8 ounces sour cream
Directions:
1. Heat up a saucepan with the ghee over medium-high warmth, add chicken pieces, season with salt and pepper, stir, diminish heat, then stew for 10 minutes.
2. Uncover the saucepan, turn chicken pieces and cook them covered again for 10 minutes more.
3. Add green onions, mix, and cook for 2 minutes more.
4. Take off warmth, add more salt and pepper if necessary, add sour cream, mix well, stir, and leave aside for 5 minutes.
5. Mix once more, separatedish onto plates and serve.
Relax and enjoy!
Nourishment: calories 200, Grams: fat 7, fiber 2, carbs 1, protein 8.

Chicken Stuffed Mushrooms

Prep & Cooking time: 20 minutes
Servings: 6
Ingredients:
• 16 ounces mushroom caps
• 4 ounces cream cheddar
• ¼ cup carrot, sliced
• 1 teaspoon farm-style sauce
• 4 tablespoons hot sauce
• ¾ cup blue cheddar sliced
• ¼ cup red onion, sliced
• ½ cup chicken meat well-cooked and sliced
• Salt and black pepper to taste

• Cooking oil

Directions:

1. In a bowl, blend cream cheddar with blue cheddar, hot sauce, farm sauce, salt, pepper, chicken, carrot, and red onion; and mix.

2. Stuff each mushroom cap with this blend, place them all on a lined preparing sheet, splash with cooking oil, put into the oven at 425 degrees F, and prepare for 10 minutes.

3. Divide onto plates and serve them.

Relax and enjoy!

Nourishment: calories 200, Grams: fat 4, fiber 1, carbs 2, protein 7.

Chicken Stuffed Avocado

Prep & Cooking time: 10 minutes

Servings: 2

Ingredients:

• 2 avocados, cut in equal parts and pitted
• ¼ cup mayonnaise
• 1 teaspoon thyme, dried
• 2 tablespoons cream cheddar
• 1 and ½ cups chicken, cooked and grated
• Salt and black pepper to taste
• ¼ teaspoon cayenne pepper
• ½ teaspoon onion powder
• ½ teaspoon garlic powder
• 1 teaspoon paprika
• Salt and black pepper to taste
• 2 tablespoons lemon juice

Directions:

1. Scoop the inner parts of your avocado halves and put it in a bowl.

2. Leave avocado shells aside for the present.

3. Add chicken to avocado flesh and mix.

4. Additionally, add mayo, thyme, cream cheddar, cayenne, onion, garlic, paprika, salt, pepper, and lemon squeeze. Mix well.

5. Stuff avocados with chicken blend, and serve.

Relax and enjoy!

Nourishment: calories 230, Grams: fat 40, fiber 11, carbs 5, protein 24.

Delectable Balsamic Chicken

Prep & Cooking time: 30 minutes
Servings: 4
Ingredients:
• 3 tablespoons coconut oil
• 2 pounds chicken breasts, skinless and boneless
• 3 garlic cloves, minced
• Salt and black pepper to taste
• 1 cup chicken stock
• 3 tablespoons stevia
• ½ cup balsamic vinegar
• 1 tomato, daintily cut
• 6 mozzarella cuts
• Some chopped basil for serving.
Directions:
1. Heat up a dish with the oil over medium-high warmth, add chicken pieces, season with salt and pepper, cook until they brown on both sides, and decrease heat.
2. Add garlic, vinegar, stock, and stevia; mix, increase heat again and cook for 10 minutes.
3. Move chicken breasts to a lined heating tray, arrange mozzarella cuts on top, at that point top with basil.
4. Cook in the grill over medium warmth until cheddar melts, and afterwards organize tomato slices over chicken pieces.
5. Dish onto plates and serve.
Relax and enjoy!
Nourishment: calories 240, Grams: fat 12, fiber 1, carbs 4, protein 27.

Vegetables

Portobello Mushroom Pizza

Prep & Cooking Time: 20 minutes
Servings: 4
Ingredients:
- 4 large portobello mushrooms, stems removed
- ¼ cup olive oil
- 1 teaspoon minced garlic
- 1 medium tomato, cut into 4 slices
- 2 teaspoons chopped fresh basil
- 1 cup shredded mozzarella cheese

Directions:
1. Preheat the oven to grill. Line a baking sheet with aluminum foil and set aside.
2. In a small bowl, toss the mushroom caps with the olive oil until well coated. Use your fingertips to rub the oil in without breaking the mushrooms.
3. Place the mushrooms on the baking sheet, gill-side down, and grill the mushrooms until they are tender on the tops, about 2 minutes.
4. Flip the mushrooms over and grill 1 minute more.
5. Take the baking sheet out and spread the garlic over each mushroom, top each with a tomato slice, sprinkle with the basil, and top with the cheese.
6. Grill the mushrooms until the cheese is melted and bubbly, about 1 minute.
7. Serve.

Nutrition -Calories: 251 Grams - Fat: 20g Protein: 14g Carbs: 7g Fiber: 3g Net Carbs: 4g

Garlicky Green Beans

Prep & Cooking Time: 20 minutes
Servings: 4

Ingredients:

- 1 pound green beans, stemmed
- 2 tablespoons olive oil
- 1 teaspoon minced garlic
- Sea salt
- Freshly ground black pepper
- ¼ cup freshly grated Parmesan cheese

Directions:

1. Preheat the oven to 425°F. Line a baking sheet with aluminum foil and set aside.
2. In a large bowl, toss together the green beans, olive oil, and garlic until well mixed.
3. Season the beans lightly with salt and pepper.
4. Spread the beans on the baking sheet and roast them until they are tender and lightly browned, stirring them once, about 10 minutes.
5. Serve topped with the Parmesan cheese.

Nutrition - Calories: 104 Grams - Fat: 9g Protein: 4g Carbs: 2g Fiber: 1g Net Carbs: 1g

Sautéed Asparagus With Walnuts

Prep & Cooking Time: 15 minutes
Servings: 4
Ingredients:

- 1½ tablespoons olive oil
- ¾ pound asparagus, woody ends trimmed
- Sea salt
- Freshly ground pepper
- ¼ cup chopped walnuts

Directions:

1. Place a large frying-pan over medium-high heat and add the olive oil.
2. Sauté the asparagus until the spears are tender and lightly browned, about 5 minutes.
3. Season the asparagus with salt and pepper.

4. Remove the frying-pan from the heat and toss the asparagus with the walnuts.
5. Serve.

Nutrition - Calories: 124 Grams - Fat: 12g Protein: 3g Carbs: 4g Fiber: 2g Net Carbs: 2g

Brussels Sprouts Casserole

Prep & Cooking Time: 45 minutes
Servings: 8
Ingredients:

- 8 bacon slices
- 1 pound Brussels sprouts, blanched for 10 minutes and cut into quarters
- 1 cup shredded Swiss cheese, divided
- ¾ cup heavy (whipping) cream

Directions:

1. Preheat the oven to 400°F.
2. Place a frying-pan over medium-high heat and cook the bacon until it is crispy, which will take about 6 minutes.
3. Reserve 1 tablespoon of bacon fat to grease the casserole dish, and roughly chop the cooked bacon.
4. Lightly oil a casserole dish with the reserved bacon fat, and set aside.
5. In a medium bowl, toss the Brussels sprouts with the chopped bacon and ½ cup of cheese and transfer the mixture to the casserole dish.
6. Pour the heavy cream over the Brussels sprouts and top the casserole with the remaining ½ cup of cheese.
7. Bake until the cheese is melted and lightly browned, and the vegetables are cooked, which should be about 20 minutes.
8. Serve.

Nutrition - Calories: 299 Grams - Fat: 11g Protein: 12g Carbs: 7g Fiber: 3g Net Carbs: 4g

Creamed Spinach

Prep & Cooking Time: 40 minutes

Servings: 4
Ingredients:
- 1 tablespoon butter
- ½ sweet onion, very thinly sliced
- 4 cups spinach, stemmed and thoroughly washed
- ¾ cup heavy (whipping) cream
- ¼ cup Herbed Chicken Stock
- Pinch sea salt
- Pinch freshly ground black pepper
- Pinch ground nutmeg

Directions:
1. In a large frying-pan over medium heat, add the butter.
2. Sauté the onion until it is lightly caramelized, about 5 minutes.
3. Stir in the spinach, heavy cream, chicken stock, salt, pepper, and nutmeg.
4. Sauté until the spinach is wilted, about 5 minutes.
5. Continue cooking the spinach until it is tender and the sauce is thickened, about 15 minutes.
6. Serve immediately.

Nutrition- Calories: 195 Grams - Fat: 20g Protein: 3g Carbs: 3g Fiber: 2g Net Carbs: 1g

Cheesy Mashed Cauliflower

Prep & Cooking Time: 20 minutes
Servings: 4
Ingredients:
- 1 head cauliflower, chopped roughly
- ½ cup shredded Cheddar cheese
- ¼ cup heavy (whipping) cream
- 2 tablespoons butter, at room temperature
- Sea salt
- Freshly ground black pepper

Directions:
1. Place a large saucepan filled three-quarters full with water over high heat and bring to a boil.

2. Blanch the cauliflower until tender, about 5 minutes, and drain.
3. Transfer the cauliflower to a food processor and add the cheese, heavy cream, and butter. Purée until very creamy and whipped.
4. Season with salt and pepper.
5. Serve.

Nutrition - Calories: 183 Grams - Fat: 15g Protein: 8g Carbs: 6g Fiber: 2g Net Carbs: 4g

Sautéed Crispy Zucchini

Prep & Cooking Time: 25 minutes
Servings: 4
Ingredients:

- 2 tablespoons butter
- 4 zucchini, cut into ¼-inch-thick rounds
- ½ cup freshly grated Parmesan cheese
- Freshly ground black pepper

Directions:

1. Place a large frying-pan over medium-high heat and melt the butter.
2. Add the zucchini and sauté until tender and lightly browned, about 5 minutes.
3. Spread the zucchini evenly in the frying-pan and sprinkle the Parmesan cheese over the vegetables.
4. Cook without stirring until the Parmesan cheese is melted and crispy where it touches the frying-pan, about 5 minutes.
5. Serve.

Nutrition- Calories: 94 Grams - Fat: 8g Protein: 4g Carbs: 1g Fiber: 1g Net Carbs: 1g

Mushrooms With Camembert

Prep & Cooking Time: 20 minutes
Servings: 4
Ingredients:

- 2 tablespoons butter
- 2 teaspoons minced garlic
- 1 pound button mushrooms, halved
- 4 ounces Camembert cheese, diced
- Freshly ground black pepper

Directions:

1. Place a large frying-pan over medium-high heat and melt the butter.
2. Sauté the garlic until translucent, about 3 minutes.
3. Sauté the mushrooms until tender, about 10 minutes.
4. Stir in the cheese and sauté until melted, about 2 minutes.
5. Season with pepper and serve.

Nutrition - Calories: 161 Grams - Fat: 13g Protein: 9g Carbs: 4g Fiber: 1g Net Carbs: 3g

Pesto Zucchini Noodles

Prep & Cooking Time: 25 minutes
Servings: 4
Ingredients:

- 4 small zucchini, ends trimmed
- ¾ cup Herb Kale Pesto
- ¼ cup grated or shredded Parmesan cheese

Directions:

1. Use a spiralizer or peeler to cut the zucchini into "noodles" and place them in a medium bowl.
2. Add the pesto and the Parmesan cheese and toss to coat.
3. Serve.

Nutrition - Calories: 93 Grams - Fat: 8g Protein: 4g Carbs: 2g Fiber: 1g Net Carbs: 2g

Artichoke and Avocado Pasta Salad

Prep & Cooking Time: 45 minutes
Servings: 10 servings
Ingredients:

- Two cups of spiral pasta (uncooked) (you could use vegetable pasta if available)
- A quarter cup of Romano cheese (grated)
- One can (fourteen oz.) of artichoke hearts (coarsely chopped and drained well)
- One avocado (medium-sized, ripe, cubed)
- Two plum tomatoes (chopped coarsely)

For the dressing:
- One tbsp. of fresh cilantro (chopped)
- Two tbsps. of lime juice
- A quarter cup of canola oil (rapeseed)
- One and a half tsps. of lime zest (grated)
  Half a tsp. each of
- Pepper (freshly ground)
- Kosher salt (coarse salt if this is not available)

Directions:
1. Follow the directions mentioned on the package for cooking the pasta. Drain them well and rinse using cold water.
2. Then, take a large-sized bowl and in it, add the pasta along with the tomatoes, artichoke hearts, cheese, and avocado. Combine them well. Then, take another bowl and add all the ingredients of the dressing to it. Whisk them together and, once combined, add the dressing over the pasta.
3. Gently toss the mixture to coat everything evenly in the dressing, and then refrigerate.

Nutrition - Calories: 188 Grams - Protein: 6g Fat: 10g Carbs: 21g Fiber: 2g

Apple, Rocket and Turkey Salad in a Jar

Prep & Cooking Time: 20 minutes
Servings: 4 servings
Ingredients:
- Three tbsps. of red wine vinegar
- Two tbsps. of chives (freshly minced)
- Half a cup of orange juice

- One to three tbsps. of sesame oil
- A quarter tsp. each of
- Pepper (coarsely ground)
- Salt

For the salad:
- Four tsps. of curry powder
  Four cups each of
- Turkey (cubed, cooked)
- Baby spinach or fresh arugula/rocket
- A quarter tsp. of salt
- Half a tsp. of pepper (coarsely ground)
- One cup of halved green grapes
- One apple (large-sized, chopped)
- Eleven oz. of mandarin oranges (properly drained)
- One tbsp. of lemon juice
  Half a cup each of
- Walnuts (chopped)
- Dried cranberries or pomegranate seeds

Directions:

1. Take a small-sized bowl and, in it, add the first 6 ingredients from the list. Whisk them. Then take a large bowl and in it, add the turkey; then add the seasonings on top of it. Toss the turkey cubes to coat them with the seasoning. Take another bowl and in it, add the lemon juice and toss the apple chunks in the juice.

2. Take four jars and divide the layers in the order I mention here - first goes the orange juice mixture, the second layer is that of the turkey, then apple, oranges, grapes, cranberries or pomegranate seeds, walnuts, and spinach/arugula. Cover the jars and then refrigerate them.

Nutrition - Calories: 471 Grams - Protein: 45g Fat: 19g Carbs: 33g Fiber: 5g.

Summertime Slaw

Prep & Cooking Time: 50 minutes
Servings: 10-12 servings
Ingredients:

- One-third cup of canola or other oil
  Three-quarter cups each of
- White vinegar
- Sugar
  One tsp. each of
- Pepper
- Salt
- One tbsp. of water
- Half a tsp. of red pepper flakes (crushed and optional)
- Two tomatoes (medium-sized, seeded, peeled, and chopped)
- One pack of coleslaw mix (fourteen oz.)
- One sweet red pepper (small-sized, chopped)
- One green pepper (small-sized, chopped)
- One onion (large-sized, chopped)
- Half a cup of sweet pickle relish

Directions:

1. Take a saucepan of large size and in it, combine water, sugar, oil, vinegar, pepper, salt, and if you want, then red pepper flakes too. Cook them over medium heat by continuously stirring the mixture. Keep stirring until it comes to a boil. Cook for another two minutes or so and make sure that all the sugar has dissolved. Once done, cool the mixture to room temperature by stirring it.

2. Take a salad bowl of large size and in it, combine the pickle relish, coleslaw mix, peppers, onion, and tomatoes. On top of the mixture, add the dressing and toss the mixture to coat it properly. Cover the mixture and put it in the refrigerator for a night.

Nutrition - Calories: 138 Grams - Protein: 1g Fat: 6g Carbs: 21g Fiber: 2g.

Zucchini and Tomato Spaghetti

Prep & Cooking Time: 30 minutes
Servings: 4 servings
Ingredients:

- Two large-sized zucchini nicely spiralized
- Three cups of red and yellow cherry tomatoes
- Four oz. of spaghetti (whole wheat – optional)
- Toppings – grated parmesan

For the avocado sauce:

- A quarter cup of olive oil
- One avocado
- Half a cup of parsley (fresh)
- Half a tsp. of salt
- Three to four green onions (only the green parts)
- One lemon (juiced)
- One clove of garlic
- A pinch of pepper (freshly ground)

Directions:

1. Firstly, take all the ingredients of the sauce and beat them so that they are combined well and form a smooth mixture. Set it aside.
2. Then, follow the directions mentioned in the package for cooking the spaghetti. Drain the cooked spaghetti and keep it aside too.
3. Take a large-sized frying-pan and heat the cherry tomatoes in it. Use a bit of olive oil. Keep cooking the tomatoes until they seem well-roasted, and they will also seem loosened with their skins split. Once done, remove the tomatoes from the flame and set them aside.
4. Then, add the zucchini to the same frying-pan. Stir and toss them for about two minutes until they look crisp. Then, add the avocado sauce and the spaghetti. Keep tossing until everything has properly combined. Season with pepper and salt as per taste. Top with parmesan and the tomatoes that you had reserved earlier.

Nutrition - Calories: 330 Grams - Protein: 7.1g Fat: 20g Carbs: 35.3g
Fiber: 8g.

White Bean Salad

Prep & Cooking Time: 15 minutes
Servings: 4 servings
Ingredients:
For the salad:

- Two green peppers, coarsely chopped
  Half a cup each of
- Chopped cucumber
- Chopped tomatoes
- One and a half cups of white beans (boiled)
  A quarter cup each of
- Green onions (chopped)
- Fresh dill (chopped)
- Parsley (chopped)
- Four eggs (hard-boiled)

For the dressing:

- One tbsp. of lemon juice
- One tsp. of vinegar
- Two tbsps. of olive oil
- One tsp. of sumac
- Half a tsp. of salt For quick onion pickle:
  One tsp. each of
- Sumac
- Salt
- Vinegar
- One tbsp. of lemon juice
- Two thinly sliced red onions (medium-sized)
- Two cups of water (hot)

Directions:

1. Take a large-sized bowl and add all the salad ingredients in it,
   but keep the eggs aside.

2. In case you do not want to pickle the onions, you can simply make thin slices and then mix them with the other ingredients. But, if you do want to pickle the onions, then continue with it before you move on to the dressing.

3. Take all the ingredients of the dressing together in one bowl and whisk them together. Then, drizzle the dressing over the salad. Toss well, and on the top, place halved eggs.

For the pickled onions:

1. First, take very hot water and place the sliced onions in it. Blanch the onions for one minute and then immediately transfer them into a pot of very cold water so that the cooking stops. Let them stay in that pot of cold water for a few minutes. Once done, drain them well.

2. Mix sumac, lemon juice, salt, and vinegar, and then pour the mixture over the onion that you just drained. Keep it for five to ten minutes. Then, add the onions into the mixture of salad and stir well. Keep some onions aside so that you can use them as a topping.

Nutrition - Calories: 449 Grams - Protein: 23.6g Fat: 23.3g Carbs: 39.7g.

Lentil Bolognese

Prep & Cooking Time: 60 minutes
Servings: 4-6 servings
Ingredients:

- Two boxes of veggie pasta, e.g. chickpea pasta
- One onion (medium-sized, finely chopped)
- One red bell pepper (finely chopped)
- Two tbsps. of olive oil
- Two carrots (large-sized, sliced)
- Four cloves of garlic (large ones, minced)
- One tbsp. of miso
  One tsp. each of
- Pepper
- Salt
- Four cups of water

- One can of tomato paste (measuring five and a half ounces)
  One cup each of
- Brown lentils (dried)
- Cherry tomatoes (halved)
- Toppings (optional) – black pepper, sage leaves, parmesan (grated)

Directions:

1. Take a large-sized frying-pan and start by heating the oil in it on medium flame. Then, add the chopped onions. In about five minutes, they will soften and appear to be translucent. Then, add the red pepper, carrots, sugar, and sea salt to the frying-pan and keep cooking. Stir the mixture from time to time. In fifteen minutes, everything will be well caramelized. Then, add the tomato paste and the garlic and let the mixture cook for three minutes or until you get a caramelized fragrance from the paste.

2. Then, add the lentils, miso, and water to the frying-pan and bring the mixture to a boil. Once the mixture is boiling, reduce the flame and keep the frying-pan uncovered while the lentils are cooking. This will take about twenty-five to thirty minutes. Keep stirring the lentils from time to time, and in case they look dry, add some water. After that, add the cherry tomatoes and keep stirring.

3. While you are cooking the lentils, take a large pot and fill it with water. Add generous amounts of salt and bring the water to a boil. Then, add the chickpea pasta into the water and cook it for about five to six minutes or until al dente. Don't overcook it. Once done, drain the water and set it aside to cool.

4. Divide the penne into four to six meal prep containers and top with Bolognese. Sprinkle a few sage leaves or a bit of parmesan if you want.

Nutrition - Calories: 486 Grams - Protein: 29.3g Fat: 9g Carbs: 78.2g Fiber: 15g.

Smoothies recipes

Almond Smoothie

Preparation Time: 20 minutes
Servings: 2
Ingredients:
- ¾ cup almonds, chopped
- ½ cup heavy whipping cream
- 2 teaspoons butter, melted
- ¼ teaspoon organic vanilla extract
- 7–8 drops liquid stevia
- 1 cup unsweetened almond milk
- ¼ cup of ice cubes

Directions:
1. In a blender, put all the listed ingredients and blend until creamy.
2. Pour the smoothie into two glasses and serve immediately.

Nutrition - Calories 365 Grams: Net Carbs 4.5 g Total Fat 34.55 g Saturated Fat 10.8 g Cholesterol 51 mg Sodium 129 mg Total Carbs 9.5 g Fiber 5 g Sugar 1.6 g Protein 8.7 g

Mocha Smoothie

Preparation Time: 20 minutes
Servings: 2
Ingredients:
- 2 teaspoons instant espresso powder
- 2–3 tablespoons granulated erythritol (sweetener)
- 2 teaspoons cocoa powder
- ½ cup plain Greek yogurt
- 1 cup unsweetened almond milk
- 1 cup of ice cubes

Directions:

1. In a blender, put all the listed ingredients and blend until creamy.
2. Pour the smoothie into two glasses and serve immediately.

Nutrition: Calories 70 Grams: Net Carbs 5.5 g Total Fat 2.8 g Saturated Fat 1 g Cholesterol 4 mg Sodium 133 mg Total Carbs 6.5 g Fiber 1 g Sugar 4.3 g   Protein 4.4 g

Strawberry Smoothie

Preparation Time: 20 minutes
Servings: 2
Ingredients:
- 4 ounces of frozen strawberries
- 2 teaspoons granulated erythritol
- ½ teaspoon organic vanilla extract
- 1/3 cup heavy whipping cream
- 1¼ cups unsweetened almond milk
- ½ cup of ice cubes

Directions:
1. In a blender, put all the listed ingredients and blend until creamy.
2. Pour the smoothie into two glasses and serve immediately.

Nutrition: Calories 115 Grams: Net Carbs 4.5 g Total Fat 9.8 g Saturated Fat 4.8 g Cholesterol 27 mg Sodium 121 mg Total Carbs 6.3 g Fiber 1.8 g Sugar 2.9 g Protein 1.4 g

Raspberry Smoothie

Preparation Time: 20 minutes
Servings: 2
Ingredients:
- ¾ cup fresh raspberries
- 3 tablespoons heavy whipping cream
- 1/3-ounce cream cheese
- 1 cup unsweetened almond milk
- ½ cup of ice cubes, crushed

Directions:
1. In a blender, put all the listed ingredients and blend until creamy.
2. Pour the smoothie into two glasses and serve immediately.

Nutrition: Calories 138 Grams: Net Carbs 3.8 g Total Fat 12 g Saturated Fat 6.4 g Cholesterol 36 mg Sodium 115 mg Total Carbs 7.3 g Fiber 3.5 g Sugar 2.1 g Protein 1.9 g

Pumpkin Smoothie

Preparation Time: 20 minutes
Servings: 2
Ingredients:

- ½ cup homemade pumpkin purée
- 4 ounces cream cheese, softened
- ¼ cup heavy cream
- ½ teaspoon pumpkin pie spice
- ¼ teaspoon ground cinnamon
- 8 drops liquid stevia
- 1 teaspoon organic vanilla extract
- 1 cup unsweetened almond milk
- ¼ cup of ice cubes

Directions:
1. In a blender, put all the listed ingredients and blend until creamy.
2. Pour the smoothie into two glasses and serve immediately.

Nutrition: Calories 296 Grams: Net Carbs 5.4 g Total Fat 27.1 g Saturated Fat 16.1g Cholesterol 83 mg Sodium 266 mg Total Carbs 8 g Fiber 2.6 g Sugar 2.4 g Protein 5.6 g

Spinach & Avocado Smoothie

Preparation Time: 20 minutes
Servings: 2
Ingredients:

- ½ large avocado, peeled, pitted, and roughly chopped

- 2 cups fresh spinach
- 1 tablespoon MCT oil
- 1 teaspoon organic vanilla extract
- 6–8 drops liquid stevia
- 1½ cups unsweetened almond milk
- ½ cup of ice cubes

Directions:

1. In a blender, put all the listed ingredients and blend until creamy.
2. Pour the smoothie into two glasses and serve immediately.

Nutrition: Calories 180 Grams: Net Carbs 10 g Total Fat 18 g Saturated Fat 9 g Cholesterol 0 mg Sodium 161 mg Total Carbs 6.5 g Fiber 4.3 g Sugar 0.6 g Protein 2.4 g

Matcha Smoothie

Preparation Time: 20 minutes
Servings: 2
Ingredients:

- 2 tablespoons chia seeds
- 2 teaspoons matcha green tea powder
- ½ teaspoon fresh lemon juice
- ½ teaspoon xanthan gum
- 10 drops liquid stevia
- 4 tablespoons plain Greek yogurt
- 1½ cups unsweetened almond milk
- ¼ cup of ice cubes

Directions:

1. In a blender, put all the listed ingredients and blend until creamy.
2. Pour the smoothie into two glasses and serve immediately.

Nutrition: Calories 85 Grams: Net Carbs 3.5 g Total Fat 5.5 g Saturated Fat 0.8 g Cholesterol 2 mg Sodium 174 mg Total Carbs 7.6 g Fiber 4.1 g Sugar 2.2 g Protein 4 g

Creamy Spinach Smoothie

Preparation Time: 20 minutes
Servings: 2
Ingredients:

- 2 cups fresh baby spinach
- 1 tablespoon almond butter
- 1 tablespoon chia seeds
- 1/8 teaspoon ground cinnamon
- Pinch of ground cloves
- ½ cup heavy cream
- 1 cup unsweetened almond milk
- ½ cup of ice cubes

Directions:

1. In a blender, put all the listed ingredients and blend until creamy.
2. Pour the smoothie into two glasses and serve immediately.

Nutrition: Calories 195 Grams: Net Carbs 2.8 g Total Fat 18.8 g Saturated Fat 7.5 g Cholesterol 41 mg   Sodium 126 mg Total Carbs 6.1 g Fiber 3.3 g Sugar 0.5 g Protein 4.5 g

Chocolate-Vanilla Almond Milk (soy, nuts)

Prep & Cooking Time:105 minutes
Servings: 1
Ingredients:

- 2 tbsp. coconut oil
- 1½ cups unsweetened almond milk
- ½ vanilla stick (crushed)
- 1 scoop organic soy protein powder (chocolate flavor)
- 4-6 drops stevia sweetener
- Optional: ½ tsp. cinnamon
- Optional: 1-2 ice cubes

Directions:

1. Add all the listed ingredients to a blender—except the ice—but including the optional cinnamon if desired.

114

2. Blend the ingredients for 1 minute; then if desired, add the optional ice cubes and blend for another 30 seconds.
3. Transfer the milk to a large cup or shaker, top with some additional cinnamon, serve, and enjoy!
4. Alternatively, store the smoothie in an airtight container or a mason jar, keep it in the fridge, and consume within 3 days. Store for a maximum of 30 days in the freezer and thaw at room temperature.

Nutrition: Calories: 422 kcal Grams: Net Carbs: 1.3 g. Fat: 34.8 g. Protein: 25.5 g. Fiber: 2.7 g. Sugar: 0.8 g.

Nutty Protein Shake (soy, peanuts, nuts)

Preparation Time: 10 minutes
Servings: 1
Ingredients:
- 2 tbsp. coconut oil
- 2 cups unsweetened almond milk
- 2 tbsp. peanut butter
- 1 scoop organic soy protein powder (chocolate flavor)
- 2-4 ice cubes
- 4-6 drops stevia sweetener

- Optional: 1 tsp. cocoa powder

Directions:
1. Add all the above-listed ingredients—except the optional ingredients—to a blender, and blend for 2 minutes.
2. Transfer the shake to a large cup or shaker. If desired, top the shake with the optional cocoa powder.
3. Stir before serving, and enjoy!
4. Alternatively, store the smoothie in an airtight container or a mason jar, keep it in the fridge, and consume within 3 days. Store for a maximum of 30 days in the freezer and thaw at room temperature.

Nutrition: Calories: 618 kcal Grams: Net Carbs: 4.4 g. Fat: 51.3 g. Protein: 34 g. Fiber: 4.9 g. Sugar: 3 g.

Chia & Coco Shake (soy, peanuts)

Preparation Time: 10 minutes
Servings: 1
Ingredients:

- 1 tbsp. chia seeds
- 6 tbsp. water
- 1 cup of coconut milk
- 2 tbsp. peanut butter
- 1 tbsp. MCT oil (or coconut oil)
- 1 scoop organic soy protein powder (chocolate flavor)
- Pinch of Himalayan salt
- 2-4 ice cubes or ½ cup of water

Directions:

1. Mix the chia seeds and 6 tablespoons of water in a small bowl; let it sit for at least 30 minutes.
2. Transfer the soaked chia seeds and all other listed ingredients to a blender and blend for 2 minutes.
3. Transfer the shake to a large cup or shaker, serve, and enjoy!
4. Alternatively, store the smoothie in an airtight container or a mason jar, keep it in the fridge, and consume within 3 days. Store for a maximum of 30 days in the freezer and thaw at room temperature.

Nutrition: Calories: 593 kcal Grams: Net Carbs: 7.4 g. Fat: 45.6 g. Protein: 36 g. Fiber: 13.9 g. Sugar: 3 g.

Dessert

Raspberry Pudding Surprise

Preparation Time: 40 minutes
Servings: 1
Ingredients
- 3 tbsp. chia seeds
- ½ cup unsweetened almond milk
- 1 scoop chocolate protein powder
- ¼ cup raspberries, fresh or frozen
- 1 tsp. honey

Directions
1. Combine the almond milk, protein powder, and chia seeds.
2. Let the mixture rest for 5 minutes before stirring.
3. Refrigerate for 30 minutes.
4. Top with raspberries.
5. Serve!

Nutritional value per **one** serving: 225 cal., 21g fat, 3g protein & 3g carbs

Vanilla Bean Dream

Preparation Time: 35 minutes
Servings: 1

Ingredients
- ½ cup extra virgin coconut oil, softened
- ½ cup coconut butter, softened
- Juice of 1 lemon
- Seeds from ½ a vanilla bean

117

1. Whisk the ingredients in an easy-to-pour cup.
2. Pour into a lined cupcake or loaf pan.
3. Refrigerate for 20 minutes. Top with lemon zest.
4. Serve!

Nutritional value per **one** serving: 205 cal., 18g fat, 7g protein & 7g carbs

White Chocolate Berry Cheesecake

Preparation Time: 5-10 minutes
Servings: 4
Ingredients

- 8 oz cream cheese, softened
- 2 oz heavy cream
- ½ tsp. Splenda
- 1 tsp. raspberries
- 1 tbsp. Da Vinci Sugar-Free syrup, white chocolate flavor

Directions

1. Whip together the ingredients to a thick consistency.
2. Divide into cups. Refrigerate. Serve!

Nutritional value per **one** serving: 330 cal., 29g fat, 6g protein & 6g carbs

Coconut Pillow

Preparation Time: 1-2 days
Servings: 4
Ingredients

- 1 can unsweetened coconut milk
- Berries of choice
- Dark chocolate, grated

Directions

1. Refrigerate the coconut milk for 24 hours.
2. Remove it from your refrigerator and whip for 2-3 minutes.
3. Fold in the berries. Season with the chocolate shavings.

4. Serve!

Nutritional value per **one** serving: 50 cal., 5g fat, 1g protein & 2g carbs

Coffee Surprise

Preparation Time: 5 minutes
Servings: 1
Ingredients

- 2 heaped tbsp. flaxseed, ground
- 100ml cooking cream
- ½ tsp. cocoa powder, dark and unsweetened
- 1 tbsp. goji berries
- Freshly brewed coffee

Directions

1. Mix the flaxseeds, cream and cocoa, and coffee.
2. Season with goji berries.
3. Serve!

Nutritional value per **one** serving: 55 cal., 45g fat, 15g protein & 3g carbs

Chocolate Cheesecake

Preparation Time: 60 minutes
Servings: 4

Ingredients

- 4 oz cream cheese
- ½ oz heavy cream
- 1 tsp. Stevia Glycerite
- 1 tsp. Splenda
- 1 oz Enjoy Life mini chocolate chips

Directions

1. Combine all the ingredients except the chocolate, to a thick consistency.
2. Fold in the chocolate chips.
3. Refrigerate in serving cups.
4. Serve!

Nutritional value per **one** serving: 230 cal., 22g fat, 6g protein & 9g carbs.

Almond Crusty

Prep + Cooking Time: 60 minutes
Servings: 4

Ingredients
- 1 cup keto almond flour
- 4 tsp. melted butter
- 2 large eggs
- ½ tsp. salt

Directions
1. Mix the almond flour and butter.
2. Add in the eggs and salt, and combine well to form a dough ball.
3. Place the dough between two pieces of parchment paper. Roll out to 10" by 16" and ¼ inch thick.
4. Bake for 30 minutes at 350°F, or until golden brown.
5. Serve!

Nutritional value per **one** serving: 190 cal., 18g fat, 8g protein & 5g carbs.

Chocolate Peanut Butter Cups

Preparation Time: 70 minutes
 Servings: 2

Ingredients
- 1 stick unsalted butter
- 1 oz / 1 cube unsweetened chocolate

- 5 packets Stevia in the Raw
- 1 tbsp. heavy cream
- 4 tbsp. peanut butter

Directions

1. In a microwave, melt the butter and chocolate.
2. Add the Stevia.
3. Stir in the cream and peanut butter.
4. Line the muffin tins. Fill the muffin cups.
5. Freeze for 60 minutes.
6. Serve!

Nutritional value per **one** serving: 175 cal., 17g fat, 2g protein & 12g carbs

Macaroon Bites

Prep + Cooking Time: 30 minutes
Servings: 2

Ingredients

- 4 egg whites
- ½ tsp. vanilla
- ½ tsp. EZ-Sweet (or equivalent of 1 cup artificial sweetener)
- 4½ tsp. water
- 1 cup unsweetened coconut

Directions

1. Preheat your oven to 375°F/190°C. Combine the egg whites, liquids, and coconut.
2. Put into the oven and reduce the heat to 325°F/160°C.
3. Bake for 15 minutes. Serve!

Nutritional value per **one** serving: 125 cal., 12g fat, 2g protein & 5g carbs.

Choco-Berry Fudge Sauce

Prep + Cooking Time: 30 minutes
Servings: 2

Ingredients

- 4 oz cream cheese, softened
- 1-3.5 oz 90% cocoa chocolate Lindt bar, chopped
- ¼ cup powdered erythritol
- ¼ cup heavy cream
- 1 tbsp. Monin sugar-free raspberry syrup

Directions

1. In a large frying-pan, melt together the cream cheese and chocolate.
2. Stir in the sweetener.
3. Remove from the heat and allow to cool.
4. Once cool, mix in the cream and syrup.
5. Serve!

Nutritional value per **one** serving: 155 cal., 15g fat, 2g protein & 4g carbs.

Choco-Coconut Pudding

Prep + Cooking Time: 65 minutes |
Servings: 1
Ingredients

- 1 cup coconut milk
- 2 tbsp. cocoa powder or organic cocoa
- ½ tsp. Stevia powder extract or 2 tbsp. honey/maple syrup
- ½ tbsp. good quality gelatin
- 1 tbsp. water

Directions

1. On medium heat, combine the coconut milk, cocoa, and sweetener.
2. In a separate bowl, mix in the gelatin and water.
3. Add to the pan and stir until fully dissolved.
4. Pour into small dishes and refrigerate for 1 hour.
5. Serve!

Nutritional value per **one** serving: 225 cal., 23g fat, 4g protein & 5g carbs.

Strawberry Frozen Dessert

Preparation Time: 45 minutes
Servings: 1

Ingredients
- ½ cup sugar-free strawberry preserves
- ½ cup Stevia in the Raw or Splenda
- 2 cups Greek Yogurt
  Ice cream maker needed

Directions
1. In a food processor, purée the strawberries. Add the strawberry preserves.
2. Add the Greek yogurt and mix fully.
3. Put into the ice cream maker for 25-30 minutes.
4. Serve!

Nutritional value per **one** serving: 85 cal., 5g fat, 2g protein & 5g carbs

Berry Layer Cake

Preparation Time: 8 minutes
Servings: 1

Ingredients
- ¼ lemon pound cake
- ¼ cup whipping cream
- ½ tsp. Truvia
- 1/8 tsp. orange flavor
- 1 cup of mixed berries

Directions
1. Using a sharp knife, divide the lemon cake into small cubes.
2. Dice the strawberries.
3. Combine the whipping cream, Truvia, and orange flavor.
4. Layer the fruit, cake, and cream in a glass.
5. Serve!

Nutritional value per **one** serving: 450 cal., 35g fat, 12g protein & 5g carbs

Chocolate Pudding

Preparation Time: 50 minutes
Servings: 1

Ingredients
- 3 tbsp. chia seeds
- 1 cup unsweetened almond milk
- 1 scoop cocoa powder
- ¼ cup fresh raspberries
- ½ tsp. keto-friendly honey

Directions
1. Mix all of the ingredients in a large bowl.
2. Let it rest for 15 minutes but stir halfway through.
3. Stir again and refrigerate for 30 minutes. Garnish with raspberries.
4. Serve!

Nutritional value per **one** serving: 430 cal., 42g fat, 4g protein & 5g carbs.

Cranberry Cream Surprise

Preparation Time: 30 minutes
Servings: 2

Ingredients
- 1 cup mashed cranberries
- ½ cup Confectioner's Style Swerve (sweetener)
- 2 tsp. natural cherry flavoring
- 2 tsp. natural rum flavoring
- 1 cup of organic heavy cream

<u>Directions</u>

1. Combine the mashed cranberries, sweetener, cherry, and rum flavorings.
2. Cover and refrigerate for 20 minutes. Whip the heavy cream until soft peaks form.
3. Layer the whipped cream and cranberry mixture. Top with fresh cranberries, mint leaves, or grated dark chocolate. Serve!

Nutritional value per **one** serving: 333 cal., 24g fat, 8g protein & 4g carbs

Chapter 7:
21 Days Pre-Planned

Meal Plan. Week 1

	BREAKFAST	LUNCH	DINNER
Monday	Smooth Coconut Porridge	Chicken Jalapeno Fritters	Chicken Caprese
Tuesday	Keto Mushroom Omelet	Chipotle Beef Chili	Frying-Pan Lasagna
Wednesday	Keto Coconut Pancakes	Chicken Enchilada Soup	Cheese Stuffed Meatballs
Thursday	Baked Cheesy Egg Muffins	Salmon Avocado Devilled Egg	Garlic Chicken
Friday	Sweet or Savory Breakfast Cookies	Chicken Paprika Meatballs	Low-Carb Pasta
Saturday	Lettuce Sandwich	Zucchini Noodle Soup	Yakitori Chicken
Sunday	Cream Cheese Pancakes	Keto Cheesy Cauliflower	Garlic Butter Salmon

Meal Plan. Week 2

	BREAKFAST	LUNCH	DINNER
MONDAY	Vibrant Scrambled Eggs	Salsa Chicken	Cauliflower And Broccoli Casserole
TUESDAY	Keto Cereal	White Chicken Chili Soup	Lamb Kofta
WEDNESDAY	Keto Tuna Salad	Mexican Ground Beef With Veggies	Cabbage Casserole
THURSDAY	Keto Pancake Bites	Salmon With Pesto	Bacon-Wrapped Chicken
FRIDAY	Beefy Baked Eggs	Mushroom Soup	Buttery Chicken With Broccoli
SATURDAY	Egg Salad	Bread Rolls	Roasted Pork Belly
SUNDAY	Keto Porridge	Lamb Chops	Butter Poached Shrimp

Meal Plan. Week 3

	BREAKFAST	LUNCH	DINNER
MONDAY	Avocado And Egg Delight	Butter Chicken	Garlic Chicken
TUESDAY	Scrambled Tofu	Chicken Fajita Soup	Lamb With Kale
WEDNESDAY	Peanut Butter Cupcakes	Keto Bread Sandwich	Stuffed Avocado
THURSDAY	Classic Bacon And Eggs	Tuna Steak	Chicken Adobo
FRIDAY	Keto Smoked Salmon And Egg Butter	Zucchini And Basil Soup	Garlic Butter Salmon
SATURDAY	Coffee And Chia Pudding	Keto Pepperoni Pizza	Keto Meatloaf
SUNDAY	Asparagus And Poached Eggs	Keto Fried Chicken	Salmon With Spinach

Chapter 8:
Measurement Conversion Table

Volume Equivalents (Liquid)

US Standard	US Standard (Ounces)	Metric (Approximate)
2 tablespoons_	1 fl. oz.	30 mL
¼ cup_	2 fl. oz.	60mL
½ cup_	4 fl. oz.	120mL
1 cup_	8 fl. oz.	240 mL
1 and ½ cups_	12 fl. oz.	355 mL
2 cups/1 pint_	16 fl. oz.	475 mL
4 cups/ 1 quart_	32 fl. oz.	1 L
1 gallon_	128 fl. oz.	4L

Volume Equivalents (Dry)

US Standard	Metric (Approximate)
1/8 teaspoon_	0.5 mL
¼ teaspoon _	1 mL
½ teaspoon_	2 mL
¾ teaspoon_	4 mL
1 teaspoon_	5 mL

1 tablespoon	15 mL
¼ cup	59 mL
1/3 cup	79 mL
½ cup	118 mL
2/3 cup	156 mL
¾ cup	177 mL
1 cup	235 mL
2 cups	475 mL
3 cups	700 mL
4 cups	1 L

Oven Temperatures

Fahrenheit (F)	Celsius (C) (Approximate)
250□	120□
300□	150□
325□	165□
350□	180□
375□	190□
400□	200□
425□	220□
450□	230□

Weight Equivalents

US Standard	Metric (Approximate)
½ ounce	15 g
1 ounce	30 g
2 ounces	60 g
4 ounces	115 g
8 ounces	225 g
12 ounces	340 g
16 ounces/1 pound	455 g

Conclusion

T he ketogenic diet is often misinterpreted and taken to be a fad diet. We would like to enlighten you with this book about the health benefits of the ketogenic diet and the advantages that the keto lifestyle brings. The ketogenic diet is a very natural type of therapy that you can do at home. It is just a shuffle in your diet, with a little bit of exercise, timely food consumption, and that is it. This book gives you an honest and practical approach towards the ketogenic diet, and we hope that it is easier for you to adopt a healthy way of life by doing so little, and yet reaping so many benefits.

By pursuing the ketogenic diet, you could gain so much. You will get good health and a lean body. You will seem fitter, brighter and smarter; and hopefully, this will change the course of your life for the better. Healthy habits and eating all that's good for the body in a tastier way, is what the keto diet is all about. The cookbook is filled with amazing easy recipes that will make your daily life hassle-free. So now, you know what the keto diet can do for you!

CPSIA information can be obtained
at www.ICGtesting.com
Printed in the USA
BVHW071502290121
599098BV00004B/231